AMERICAN ACADEMY OF ORTHOPAEDIC SURGEONS

First Aid, CPR, and AED

Fourth Edition

Alton Thygerson, Ed.D.

Medical Writer

Benjamin Gulli, MD

Medical Editor

JONES AND BARTLETT PUBLISHERS

Sudbury, Massachusetts

BOSTON   TORONTO   LONDON   SINGAPORE

JONES AND BARTLETT PUBLISHERS

40 Tall Pine Drive
Sudbury, MA 01776
978-443-5000
esci@jbpub.com
http://www.SafetyCampus.org

Jones and Bartlett Publishers Canada
2406 Nikanna Road
Mississauga, ON L5C 2W6
Canada

Jones and Bartlett Publishers International
Barb House, Barb Mews
London W6 7PA
United Kingdom

Production Credits
Chief Executive Officer: Clayton Jones
Chief Operating Officer: Donald W. Jones, Jr.
President: Robert Holland
V.P., Sales and Marketing: William J. Kane
V.P., Production and Design: Anne Spencer
V.P., Manufacturing and Inventory Control: Therese Bräuer
Publisher: Lawrence D. Newell
Associate Managing Editor: Jennifer Reed
Senior Production Editor: Linda S. DeBruyn
Production Editor: Scarlett Stoppa
Text Design: Studio Montage
Typesetting: Nesbitt Graphics, Bret Kerr
Illustrations: Rolin Graphics
Interior Photos: Richard Nye
Cover Design: Kristin Ohlin
Cover Photograph: MIEMSS
Printing and Binding: Courier Company

AMERICAN ACADEMY OF ORTHOPAEDIC SURGEONS

Editorial Credits
Chief Education Officer: Mark W. Wieting
Director, Department of Publications: Marilyn L. Fox, PhD
Managing Editor: Lynne Roby Shindoll
Senior Editor: Barbara A. Scotese

The first aid, CPR, and AED procedures in this book are based on the most current recommendations of responsible medical sources. The American Academy of Orthopaedic Surgeons and the publisher, however, make no guarantee as to, and assume no responsibility for, the correctness, sufficiency, or completeness of such information or recommendations. Other or additional safety measures may be required under particular circumstances.

Library of Congress Cataloging-in-Publication Data

First Aid and CPR, Standard / American Academy of Orthopaedic Surgeons.—4th ed.
    p.   cm.
  At head of title: American Academy of Orthopaedic Surgeons.
  Includes index.
    ISBN 0-7637-2789-X (alk. paper)
  1. First aid in illness and injury.   2. CPR (First aid)   I. Thygerson, Alton J. II. American Academy of Orthopaedic Surgeons
First Aid, CPR, and AED Essentials
  ISBN 0-7637-2777-6

Additional illustrations and photo credits appear on page 143, which constitutes a continuation of the copyright page.
08 07 06 05 04   10 9 8 7 6 5 4 3 2 1

American Academy of Orthopaedic Surgeons Emergency Care and Safety Institute

Congratulations on selecting an American Academy of Orthopaedic Surgeons (AAOS) Emergency Care and Safety Institute training program! In 1971, the AAOS pioneered EMS education by publishing *Emergency Care and Transportation of the Sick and Injured*, the first EMS training program available. Today, the AAOS Emergency Care and Safety Institute continues that dedication to future emergency responders and the instructors who are paving their way.

About the AAOS

The AAOS provides education and practice management services for orthopaedic surgeons and allied health professionals. The AAOS also serves as an advocate for improved patient care and informs the public about the science of orthopaedics. Founded in 1933, the not-for-profit AAOS has grown from a small organization serving less than 500 members to the world's largest medical association of musculoskeletal specialists. The AAOS now serves about 24,000 members internationally.

About the AAOS Emergency Care and Safety Institute

The AAOS name and training programs are recognized and revered worldwide by business and industry, colleges and universities, and fire, EMS, and law enforcement agencies. The quality, affordability, and administrative ease make the AAOS Emergency Care and Safety Institute training programs appealing worldwide.

Every AAOS Emergency Care and Safety Institute textbook is the center of an integrated teaching and learning system that offers instructor, student, and technology resources to better support instructors and prepare students. The instructor supplements provide practical, hands-on, time-saving tools like PowerPoint presentations, customizable test banks, and web-based distance learning resources. The student supplements are designed to help students retain the most important information and to assist them in preparing for exams. And, a key component to the teaching and learning systems are technology resources that provide interactivities and simulations to help students become great emergency responders.

AMERICAN ACADEMY OF ORTHOPAEDIC SURGEONS

Table of Contents

Your First Aid & CPR IQ

Test your current knowledge. Read each question and place your answer in the "Pre-check" column. After reading this manual and completing your course, read the questions again and place your answers in the "Post-check" column. Compare your answers and see what you have learned.

Question	Pre-check			Post-check		
1. Most communities use 9-1-1 as their emergency telephone number.	T	F	Uncertain	T	F	Uncertain
2. Chest pain is one of the most frequent signals of a heart attack.	T	F	Uncertain	T	F	Uncertain
3. Someone coughing forcefully may be choking, and abdominal thrusts should be given.	T	F	Uncertain	T	F	Uncertain
4. Unresponsive breathing victims should be placed on their side.	T	F	Uncertain	T	F	Uncertain
5. Adult CPR requires the rescuer to give 5 chest compressions and 1 rescue breath.	T	F	Uncertain	T	F	Uncertain
6. Rescue breathing should be given to any unresponsive, non-breathing victim.	T	F	Uncertain	T	F	Uncertain
7. Open a victim's airway by tilting the head back and lifting the chin.	T	F	Uncertain	T	F	Uncertain
8. Direct pressure and elevation can control most injuries involving bleeding.	T	F	Uncertain	T	F	Uncertain
9. Heat should be applied quickly to any muscle, bone, or joint injuries to reduce swelling.	T	F	Uncertain	T	F	Uncertain
10. Applying butter is an effective treatment for first degree burns.	T	F	Uncertain	T	F	Uncertain
11. An object impaled (stuck) in the body should removed so that bleeding can be controlled.	T	F	Uncertain	T	F	Uncertain
12. A splint is something used to stabilize (reduce movement) a broken bone.	T	F	Uncertain	T	F	Uncertain
13. Most injured victims require a complete physical exam.	T	F	Uncertain	T	F	Uncertain
14. Sugar should be given to a responsive victim suspected of suffering a diabetic emergency.	T	F	Uncertain	T	F	Uncertain
15. Activated charcoal is a substance that a poison control center may ask you to administer for an ingested poisoning.	T	F	Uncertain	T	F	Uncertain
16. Ice should be applied to a snakebite wound.	T	F	Uncertain	T	F	Uncertain
17. Rub or massage a frostbitten part to quickly rewarm it.	T	F	Uncertain	T	F	Uncertain
18. Salt tablets should be given to victims of heat emergencies.	T	F	Uncertain	T	F	Uncertain
19. Hypothermia occurs only in subfreezing temperatures.	T	F	Uncertain	T	F	Uncertain
20. Extremely hot skin indicates heat exhaustion.	T	F	Uncertain	T	F	Uncertain

Background Information

Need for First Aid Training

It's better to know first aid and not need it than to need it and not know it. Everyone should be able to perform first aid because most people will eventually find themselves in a situation requiring it, either for another person or for themselves.

A delay of as little as a few minutes when a person's heart stops can mean the difference between life and death. However, most injuries do not require life-saving efforts. During their entire lifetime, most people will see only one or two situations involving life-threatening conditions. While saving lives is important, knowing what to do for less severe injuries demands greater attention and more first aid training.

What Is First Aid?

First aid is one of those things you need to know—but never want to use. *First aid* is the immediate care given to an injured or suddenly ill person ▶Table 1 . First aid does *not* take the place of proper medical treatment. Rather, it furnishes temporary assistance until the victim receives competent medical care, if needed, or until the chance for recovery without medical care is assured. Most injuries and illnesses do not require medical care.

Properly applied, first aid may mean the difference between life and death, between a rapid recovery and long hospitalization, or between temporary disability and permanent injury. First aid involves more than doing things for others; it also includes the things that people can do for themselves.

Recognizing a serious medical emergency and knowing how to get help may mean the difference between life and death. Recognition can be delayed because neither the victim nor bystanders know basic symptoms (eg, a heart attack victim may wait hours after the onset of symptoms before seeking help). Moreover, most people do not know first aid; even if they do, they may panic in an emergency.

Table 1: Leading Causes of Death	
1. Heart Disease	> 700,000
2. Cancer	> 500,000
3. Stroke	> 150,000
4. Chronic Lung Disease	> 100,000
5. Unintentional Injury	> 90,000

Legal Considerations

Fear of lawsuits has made some people reluctant about getting involved at emergency scenes. First aiders, however, are rarely sued; those who are usually receive a favorable ruling from courts.

Consent

Before giving first aid, a first aider must have the victim's consent (permission). Touching another person without his or her permission or consent is unlawful (known as battery) and could be grounds for a lawsuit. Likewise, giving first aid without the victim's consent is unlawful.

Expressed Consent

Consent must be obtained from every conscious, mentally competent (able to make a rational decision) person of legal age. Tell the victim your name and that you have first aid training, and explain what you will be doing. Permission from the victim may be expressed either with words or with a nod of the head.

Implied Consent

Implied consent involves an unresponsive victim in a life-threatening condition. It is assumed or "implied" that an unresponsive victim would consent to lifesaving help. When a child is in a life-threatening situation, and the parent or legal guardian is not available for consent, first aid should be given based on implied consent. Do not withhold first aid from a minor just to obtain parental or guardian permission.

Abandonment

Abandonment means leaving a victim after starting to give help without ensuring someone else will continue the care at the same level or higher. Once you have started providing care, you must not leave a victim who still needs first aid until another competent and trained person takes responsibility for the victim.

Negligence

Negligence means not following accepted standards of care and causing injury to the victim. Negligence involves:

1. Having a duty to act
2. Breaching that duty (by giving substandard care)
3. Causing injury and damages

Duty to Act

No one is required to render first aid when no legal duty exists. Duty to act may occur in the following situations:

- *When your employment requires it.* If your employer designates you as responsible for rendering first aid to meet OSHA (Occupational Safety and Health Administration) requirements and you are called to an injury scene, you have a duty to act. Examples of occupations with job descriptions that include a duty to act include law enforcement officers, park rangers, athletic trainers, lifeguards, and teachers. (▼Figure 1)

(Figure 1) Duty to act

- *When a pre-existing responsibility exists.* You may have a pre-existing relationship with other persons that demands you be responsible for them, which means you must give first aid if they need it. Examples include a parent for a child, or a driver for a passenger.

Duty to act means following guidelines for standards of care. Standards of care ensure quality care and protection for injured or suddenly ill victims.

Breach of Duty

Generally, a first aider breaches (breaks) his or her duty to a victim by failing to provide the type of care that would be provided by a person having the same or similar training. One's duty can be breached by acts of omission or acts of commission. An *act of omission* is the failure to do what a reasonably prudent person with the same or similar training would do in the same or similar circumstances. An *act of commission* is doing something that a reasonably prudent person would *not* do under the same or similar circumstances. Forgetting to put on a dressing is an act of omission; cutting a snakebite site is an act of commission.

Injury and Damages Inflicted

Injury or damages must have resulted from a breach of duty. In addition to physical damage, injury and damage can include physical pain and suffering, mental anguish, medical expenses, and sometimes loss of earnings and earning capacity.

Good Samaritan Laws

In most emergencies, you are not legally required to give first aid. To encourage people to assist others needing help, Good Samaritan laws grant immunity against lawsuits. Although laws vary from state to state, Good Samaritan immunity generally applies only when the rescuer is (1) acting during an emergency, (2) acting in good faith, which means he or she has good intentions, (3) acting without compensation, and (4) not guilty of any malicious misconduct or gross negligence toward the victim (deviating from all rational first aid guidelines).

Good Samaritan laws are not a substitute for competent first aid or for keeping within the scope of your training.

To find out about your state's Good Samaritan laws, ask for information at your local library or an attorney.

Meeting OSHA Guidelines

This chapter covers the following OSHA Guidelines for First Aid training:

- Section III. B. 1. Injury and acute illness as a health problem.
- Section III. B. 4. The legal aspects of providing first aid services.

[Handwritten notes at bottom of page:]

— EXPRESSED — Can / Help You

— IMPLIED — Unconscious

    — Under 18

Learning Activities

What Is First Aid?

Directions: Circle Yes if you agree with the statement, and circle No if you disagree.

Yes (No)   **1.** In most locations, an ambulance can arrive within minutes. This quick response means that most people do not need to learn first aid.

(Yes) No   **2.** Correct first aid can mean the difference between life and death.

(Yes) No   **3.** Most injuries do not require life-saving first aid efforts.

Yes (No)   **4.** You need to call for an ambulance and/or seek advanced medical care for all injured victims.

(Yes) No   **5.** In most situations, before giving first aid, you must get consent (permission) from the victim.

Yes (No)   **6.** If you ask a victim if you can help, and she says "No," you can ignore her and proceed to give first aid whether she likes it or not.

(Yes) No   **7.** Employers can designate people as first aiders. This means that they must give first aid to injured employees while on the job.

Yes (No)   **8.** First aiders who help injured victims are often sued.

(Yes) No   **9.** Good Samaritan laws provide a degree of protection for first aiders who act in a rational manner during an emergency, in good faith, and without compensation.

Scenario: You are driving slowly looking for a house number in an unfamiliar residential area. You are attempting to deliver an important package to a customer. You see an elderly woman lying at the bottom of porch stairs outside of a house. You see no one else in the neighborhood, and you are alone. You quickly, but safely, stop your vehicle in front of the victim's house. As you approach the victim, you notice that her skin appears bluish, and she is motionless.

Yes   No   **10.** Do you have to stop to help her?

_____   **11.** If you stop and help, which type of consent would apply in this case?
            A. expressed   **B.** implied

Yes   No   **12.** If she does not respond to your tapping on her shoulders and shouting "Are you O.K.?" you can leave her and assume that someone else who is more competent or is a family member will arrive shortly to help her.

Yes   No   **13.** You decide to help. You straighten one of her legs, which causes a bone to protrude through the skin. Would this increase the likelihood of being sued?

Yes   No   **14.** For the situation in number 13, the Good Samaritan law protects you from being sued.

Yes   No   **15.** If the woman were your mother under your custodial care, you must give first aid to her.

Chapter 2

Action at an Emergency

Bystander Intervention

The bystander is a vital link between the emergency medical service (EMS) and the victim. Typically it is a bystander who first recognizes a situation as an emergency and acts to help the victim. A bystander must perform the following actions quickly and reliably.

Recognize the Emergency

To help in an emergency, the bystander has to notice that something is wrong—usually a person's appearance or behavior or the surroundings suggesting something unusual has happened.

Decide to Help

At some time, everyone will have to decide whether to help another person. Making a quick decision to get involved at the time of an emergency is unlikely to occur unless the bystander has previously considered, the possibility of helping. Thus, **the most important time to make the decision to help is *before* you ever encounter an emergency.**

Deciding to help is an attitude about people, about emergencies, and about one's ability to deal with emergencies. It is an attitude that takes time to develop and is affected by a number of factors.

Call EMS, If Needed

People often make inappropriate decisions regarding calling EMS personnel. They delay calling for an ambulance until they are absolutely sure that an emergency exists, or they elect to bypass EMS personnel and transport the victim to medical care in a private vehicle. Such actions can present significant dangers to victims. Fortunately, most injuries and sudden illnesses that you will render care for will not require the need for advanced medical care—only first aid.

Assess the Victim

The bystander must decide if life-threatening conditions exist and what kind of help a victim needs immediately.

Provide Care

Often the most critical life-support measures are effective only if started immediately by the nearest available person. That person usually will be a layperson—a bystander.

Post-Care Reactions

After giving care for serious conditions, rescuers can feel an emotional "letdown," which is frequently overlooked. Discussing your feelings, fears, and reactions following the event can help prevent later emotional problems. You can talk to a trusted friend, a mental health professional, or a member of the clergy. Bringing out your feelings quickly helps to relieve personal anxieties and stress.

Scene Survey

If you are at the scene of an emergency situation, do a quick survey of the scene that includes looking for three things: (1) hazards that could be dangerous to you, the victim(s), or bystanders; (2) the cause (mechanism) of the injury or illness; and (3) the number of victims. This survey should only take a few seconds.

First, as you approach an emergency scene, scan the area for immediate dangers to yourself or to the victim. You cannot help another if you also become a victim. Always ask yourself: Is the scene safe to enter? (For details about specific hazards at an emergency scene, refer to Chapter 18.)

The second thing to do is to try to determine the cause of any injury or illness. Be sure to tell EMS personnel about your findings, so that they can fully recognize the extent of the problem.

Finally, determine how many people are involved. There may be more than one victim, so look around and ask about others involved.

Seek Medical Attention

Knowing when to call for an ambulance is important. To know when to call, you must be able to tell the difference between a minor injury or illness and a life-threatening one. For example, upper abdominal pain can be as minor as indigestion or as severe as a heart attack needing

prompt medical care. Wheezing may be related to a person's asthma, for which the person can use his or her prescribed inhaler for quick relief, or it can be as serious as a severe allergic reaction from a bee sting.

Not every cut needs stitches, nor does every burn require medical attention. It is, however, always best to err on the side of caution.

According to the American College of Emergency Physicians (ACEP), if the answer to any of the following questions is yes, or if you are unsure, call 9-1-1 or your local emergency number (if other than 9-1-1) for help.

- Is the victim's condition life-threatening?
- Could the condition get worse and become life-threatening on the way to the hospital?
- Does the victim need the skills or equipment of emergency medical technicians or paramedics?
- Would distance or traffic conditions cause a delay in getting to the hospital?

ACEP also recommends that the following conditions are warning signs that require immediate transport to the hospital emergency department, either in an ambulance or car:

- fainting
- chest or abdominal pain or pressure
- sudden dizziness, weakness, or change in vision
- difficulty breathing, shortness of breath
- severe or persistent vomiting
- sudden, severe pain anywhere in the body
- suicidal or homicidal feelings
- bleeding that does not stop after 10 to 15 minutes of pressure
- a gaping wound with edges that do not come together
- problems with movement or sensation following an injury
- cuts on the hand or face
- puncture wounds
- the possibility that foreign bodies such as glass or metal may have entered a wound
- most animal bites and all human bites
- hallucinations and clouding of thoughts
- a stiff neck in association with a fever or a headache

- a bulging or abnormally depressed fontanel (soft spot) in infants
- stupor or dazed behavior accompanying a high fever that is not alleviated by acetaminophen or aspirin
- unequal pupil size, loss of consciousness, blindness, staggering, or repeated vomiting after a head injury
- spinal injuries
- severe burns
- poisoning
- drug overdose

When a serious situation occurs, call EMS (9-1-1 in most communities) *first*. Do *not* call your doctor, the hospital, a friend, relatives, or neighbors for help before you call EMS. Calling anyone else first only wastes time.

If the situation is not an emergency, call your doctor. However, if you are in *any* doubt as to whether the situation is an emergency, call EMS.

How to Call EMS

To receive emergency assistance of every kind in most communities, you simply phone 9-1-1 (▶Figure 1). Check to see if this is true in your community. Emergency telephone numbers usually are listed on the inside front cover of telephone directories. Keep these numbers near or on every telephone. Call "0" (the operator) if you do not know the emergency number.

When you call EMS, the dispatcher will often ask for the following information. Speak slowly and clearly when you provide this information.

1. Your name and the phone number you are calling from. This prevents false calls and allows a dispatch center to call back if disconnected or for additional information if needed.

2. The victim's location. Give the address, names of intersecting roads, and other landmarks, if possible. Also, tell the specific location of the victim (eg, "in the basement").

3. What happened. State the nature of the emergency (eg, "My husband fell off a ladder and is not moving.").

4. Number of persons needing help and any special conditions.

5. Victim's condition (eg, "My husband's head is bleeding.") and any first aid you have provided (such as pressing on the site of the bleeding).

Figure 1 For help, phone 9-1-1 or the local emergency number.

Do *not* hang up the phone unless the dispatcher instructs you to do so. Enhanced 9-1-1 systems can track a call, but some communities lack this technology or are still using a seven-digit emergency number. Since cell phones cannot be tracked through enhanced 9-1-1, it is important that the number be provided to the dispatcher and that all information is conveyed. Also, the EMS dispatcher may tell you how best to care for the victim. If you send someone else to call, have the person report back to you so you can be sure the call was made.

Disease Precautions

First aiders must understand the risk of infectious diseases, which can range from mild to life threatening. The risk of getting a disease from a victim is very low. First aiders should know how to protect themselves against diseases carried by the blood and air. Precautionary measures help protect against infection from viruses and bacteria.

Bloodborne Disease

Some diseases are caused by microorganisms that are "borne" (carried) in a person's bloodstream. Contact with blood infected with such microorganisms may cause infection. Of the many bloodborne pathogens, three pose significant health threats to first aiders: hepatitis B virus (HBV), hepatitis C virus (HCV), and human immunodeficiency virus (HIV).

Hepatitis B

Hepatitis is a viral infection of the liver. Types A, B, and C are seen most often. Each is caused by a different virus.

A vaccine for hepatitis B is available and recommended for all infants and for adults who may have contact with carriers of the disease or with blood. Medical and laboratory workers, police, intravenous drug users, people with multiple sexual partners, and those living with someone who has a life-long infection are at high risk of hepatitis B (and hepatitis C as well). Vaccination is the best defense against HBV. There is no chance of developing hepatitis B from the vaccine. Federal laws require employers to offer a series of three vaccine injections free to all employees who may be at risk of exposure.

Without vaccination shots, exposure to hepatitis B may produce symptoms within two weeks to six months after the exposure. People with hepatitis B infection may be symptom free, but that does *not* mean they are not contagious. These people may infect others who are exposed to their blood. Symptoms of hepatitis B resemble those of the flu and include fatigue, nausea, loss of appetite, stomach pain, and perhaps a yellowing of the skin.

Hepatitis B starts as an inflammation of the liver and usually lasts one to two months. In a few people, the infection is very serious, and in some, mild infection continues for life. The virus may stay in the liver and can lead to severe damage (cirrhosis) and liver cancer. Medical treatment that begins immediately after exposure may prevent the infection from developing.

Hepatitis C

Hepatitis C is caused by a different virus from HBV, but both diseases have a great deal in common. Like hepatitis B, hepatitis C affects the liver and can lead to long-term liver disease and liver cancer. Hepatitis C varies in severity and there may not be any symptoms at the time of infection. Currently, there is no vaccine or effective treatment for hepatitis C.

HIV

A person infected with HIV can infect others, and HIV-infected persons almost always develop acquired immunodeficiency syndrome (AIDS), which interferes with the body's ability to fight off other diseases. No vaccine is available to prevent HIV infection, which eventually proves fatal. The best defense against AIDS is to avoid becoming infected.

Protection

In most cases, you can control the risk of exposure to bloodborne pathogens by wearing the proper Personal Protective Equipment (PPE) and by following some simple procedures.

Personal Protective Equipment (PPE)

Personal protective equipment (PPE) prevents an organism from entering the body. The most common type of protection is when a rescuer uses medical exam gloves. The Food and Drug Administration (FDA), the Centers for Disease Control and Prevention (CDC), and the Occupational Safety and Health Administration (OSHA) have stated that vinyl and latex medical exam gloves are equally protective. Some rescuers are allergic to latex, but can wear vinyl or Nitrile gloves. All first aid kits should have several pairs of medical exam gloves (▼Figure 2).

Protective eyewear and a standard surgical mask may be necessary at some emergencies; first aiders ordinarily will not have or need such equipment.

Mouth-to-barrier devices are recommended for rescue breathing and cardiopulmonary resuscitation (CPR). There are no documented cases of disease transmission to a rescuer as a result of performing unprotected CPR on an infected victim. Nevertheless, a mouth-to-barrier device should be used whenever possible (▶Figure 3).

Universal Precautions and Body Substance Isolation Techniques

Individuals infected with HBV or HIV may not show symptoms and may not even know they are infectious. For that reason, all human blood and body fluids should be considered infectious, and precautions should be taken to avoid contact. The *body substance isolation* (BSI) technique assumes that *any* body fluid is a possible risk. EMS personnel routinely follow BSI procedures, even if blood or body fluids are not visible.

(**Figure 2**) Whenever possible, use gloves as a barrier.

B. S. I.
Body Substance Isolation.

Figure 3 Pocket face mask, one-way valve

OSHA requires any company with employees who are expected to give first aid in an emergency to follow *universal precautions,* which assume that *all* blood and *certain* body fluids pose a risk for transmission of HBV and HIV. OSHA defines an employee who assists another with a nosebleed or a cut as a "Good Samaritan." Such acts, however, are not considered occupational exposure unless the employee who provided the assistance is a member of a first aid team or is designated or expected to render first aid as part of his or her job. In essence, OSHA's requirement excludes unassigned employees who perform unanticipated first aid.

Whenever there is a chance that you could be exposed to bloodborne pathogens, your employer must provide appropriate PPE, which might include eye protection, medical exam gloves, gowns, and masks. The PPE must be accessible, and your employer must provide training to help you choose the right PPE for your work.

While EMS personnel follow BSI procedures and OSHA requires designated worksite first aiders to follow universal precautions, what should a typical first aider do? It makes sense for first aiders to follow BSI procedures and assume that *all* blood and body fluids are infectious and follow appropriate protective measures.

Coping with Emergencies

When an injury occurs, first aiders can protect themselves and others against bloodborne pathogens by following these steps:

1. Wear appropriate PPE, such as gloves.
2. If you have been trained in the correct procedures, use absorbent barriers to soak up blood or other infectious materials.
3. Clean the spill area with an appropriate disinfecting solution, such as diluted bleach.
4. Discard contaminated materials in an appropriate waste disposal container.

If you have been exposed to blood or body fluids:

1. Use soap and water to wash the parts of your body that have been contaminated.
2. Report the incident to your supervisor, if the exposure happens while at work. Otherwise, contact your personal physician. Early action can prevent the development of hepatitis B and enable affected workers to track potential HIV infection.

The best protection against bloodborne disease is to use the safeguards described here. By following these guidelines, first aiders can decrease their chances of contracting bloodborne illnesses.

Airborne Disease

Infective organisms such as bacteria or viruses that are introduced into the air by coughing or sneezing are said to be "airborne." Droplets of mucus that carry those bacteria or viruses can then be inhaled by other individuals. The rate of tuberculosis (TB) has increased recently and is receiving much attention. TB, caused by bacteria, sometimes settles in the lungs and can be fatal. In most cases, a first aider will not know that a victim has TB. Assume that any person with a cough, especially one who is in a nursing home or a shelter, may have TB. Other symptoms include fatigue, weight loss, chest pain, and coughing up blood. If a surgical mask is available, wear it or wrap a handkerchief over your nose and mouth.

Meeting OSHA Guidelines

This chapter covers the following OSHA Guidelines for First Aid training:

- Section III. B. 1. Injury and acute illness as a health problem.
- Section III. B. 2. Interactions with the local emergency medical services system.
- Section III. F. 1a-f. Universal precautions: Trainees should be provided with adequate instruction on the need for and use of universal precautions.

D.O.T.S.
Deformity

Learning Activities

Action at an Emergency

Directions: Circle Yes if you agree with the statement, and circle No if you disagree.

Yes No **1.** A scene survey should be done before giving first aid to an injured victim.

Yes No **2.** For a severely injured victim, call the victim's doctor before calling for an ambulance.

Yes No **3.** Most communities use the 9-1-1 telephone number for emergencies.

Yes No **4.** First aiders should assume that blood and all body fluids are infectious.

Yes No **5.** If you are exposed to blood while on the job, report it to your supervisor, and if off the job, your personal physician.

Yes No **6.** First aid kits should contain medical exam gloves.

Scenario: You are rushing parts to one of your largest customer's broken machines. Because "time is money," the customer is losing a lot for each hour its machine is down. It's beginning to rain. Suddenly, you see a motorcyclist skid off the highway, and end up in a ditch. You have a cellular telephone in your car.

7. Name the 5 actions that a bystander can take at an emergency.

a. _____ d. _____

b. _____ e. _____

c. _____

8. A scene survey consists of looking for what three things?

a. _____

b. _____

c. _____

9. When talking with an EMS dispatcher, what 5 items should you be prepared to provide?

a. _____ d. _____

b. _____ e. _____

c. _____

10. When an injury occurs, you can protect yourself and others against bloodborne pathogens by wearing: _____

Chapter 3

Finding Out What's Wrong

Victim Assessment

Victim assessment is an important first aid skill. It requires an understanding of each assessment step as well as decision-making skills.

Every time you encounter a victim, first check out the scene. The scene survey determines the safety of the scene, the victim's cause of injury or nature of illness, and the number of victims. Without a scene survey, a potentially dangerous situation could result in further injury to the victim or to you and others.

The scene survey is followed by the initial victim assessment. During the initial victim assessment, the first aider identifies and corrects immediate life-threatening conditions involving problems with the victim's airway, breathing, and circulation (the ABCs). Victims with immediate life-threatening conditions can die within minutes unless their problems are quickly recognized and corrected. Determining the type of injury or illness is also part of the initial assessment.

A physical examination and medical history follow the initial assessment. These steps can reveal information that will help identify the injury or illness, its severity, and appropriate first aid. Detailed information is gained about the victim's injury (eg, painful ankle, bleeding nose) or chief complaint (eg, chest pain, itchy skin).

If two or more people are injured, attend to the quiet one first. A quiet victim might not be breathing or have a heartbeat. A victim who is talking, crying, or otherwise alert is obviously breathing.

Initial Assessment

The goal of the initial assessment is to determine whether there are life-threatening problems that require quick care (▶Skill Scan). This assessment involves evaluating the victim's airway (A), breathing (B), and circulation (C). The following step-by-step initial assessment should not be changed. It takes less than a minute to complete, unless first aid is required at any point. By the end of the initial assessement, the victim's problem will most likely be identified as being an injury or an illness.

Skill Scan   Initial Assessment

1. Responsive? Tap and shout.

2. A = Airway open? Head tilt-chin lift.

3. B = Breathing? Look, listen, and feel.

4. C = Circulation? Check for signs of circulation.

Check for responsiveness by speaking to the victim. If the person can talk, breathing and heartbeat are present. Ask the victim his name, if he knows where he is, and what happened. If the victim does not respond, tap his or her shoulder and ask, "Are you okay?" If there is no response, consider the victim as being unresponsive.

Immediate Threats to Life

A: Airway   21% O2

The airway must be open for breathing. If the victim is speaking or crying, the airway is open. If a responsive victim cannot talk, cry, or cough forcefully, the airway is probably obstructed and must be checked and cleared. In this case, abdominal thrusts (Heimlich maneuver) can be given to clear an obstructed airway in a responsive adult victim. This and other techniques for airway, breathing, and circulation care are described in detail in Chapter 4.

In an unresponsive victim lying face up, the most common airway obstruction is the tongue. Snoring is evidence of this. If there is no suspected spinal injury, use the head tilt–chin lift method to open the airway. If a spinal injury is likely, use the jaw-thrust method to prevent further injury. Refer to Chapter 4 for details.

Once the victim's airway is clear of obstruction, the initial assessment can continue.

B: Breathing

A breathing rate between 12 and 20 times per minute is normal for adults. Victims who are having difficulty moving air and who are breathing less than eight times per minute or more than 24 times per minute need care. Note any breathing difficulties or unusual breathing sounds such as wheezing, crowing, gurgling, or snoring. This step primarily focuses upon whether or not the victim is breathing and obvious breathing difficulties rather than the breathing rate.

Check for breathing in an unresponsive victim after opening the airway. Watch for the victim's chest to rise and fall as you place your ear next to the victim's mouth. "Look, listen, and feel" for about 10 seconds to check for breathing. If the victim is not breathing, keep the airway open and breathe two slow breaths into the victim. Refer to Chapter 4 for details. Whenever possible, use a mouth-to-barrier device (mask or face shield).

C: Circulation

After checking and correcting any airway and breathing problems, check the victim's circulation. This can be done by checking the signs of circulation—breathing, cough-

S: SEVERE BLEEDING

ing, movement, noting the skin color and temperature, and searching for severe bleeding.

Signs of Circulation The signs of normal circulation include breathing, coughing, movement, and normal skin condition.

Severe Bleeding Check for severe bleeding by looking over the victim's entire body for blood (blood-soaked clothing or blood pooling on the floor or the ground). Controlling bleeding requires the application of direct pressure or a pressure bandage. Avoid contact with the victim's blood, if possible, by using medical exam gloves or extra layers of dressings or cloth. Control any bleeding with pressure as described in Chapter 5.

Skin Condition A quick check of the victim's skin can also provide information about circulatory status. Check skin temperature, color, and condition (eg, moist, dry). Skin color, especially in light-skinned people, reflects the circulation under the skin as well as oxygen status. In darkly pigmented people, changes might not be readily apparent but can be assessed by the appearance of the nail beds, the inside of the mouth, and the inner eyelids. When the skin's blood vessels constrict or the pulse slows, the skin becomes cool and pale or cyanotic (blue-gray color). When the skin's blood vessels dilate or blood flow increases, the skin becomes warm.

You can get a rough idea of temperature by putting the back of your hand or wrist on the victim's forehead. If the victim has a fever, you should be able to feel it. Abnormal skin temperature will feel hot, cool, cold, or clammy (cool and moist).

If you suspect a spinal injury, do not move the victim. See Chapter 9 for the best way to immobilize a suspected spinal injury.

Physical Exam and SAMPLE History

The initial assessment is followed by a physical examination and the **SAMPLE** history. During this time you will note the victim's signs and symptoms:

- *Signs* = victim's conditions you can see, feel, hear or smell
- *Symptoms* = things the victim feels and is able to describe; known as the "chief complaint"

Physical Examination Check the victim's head, neck, chest, abdomen, pelvis, and extremities ▶ Skill Scan . To help you evaluate these areas, look and feel for the following signs of injury: deformities, open injuries, tenderness, and swelling. The mnemonic **D-O-T-S** is helpful in remembering the signs of injury.

Deformities occur when bones are broken, causing an

Skill Scan   Physical Exam: Injury

Briefly Look and Feel for D-O-T-S Throughout the Body

1. **Head:** Check the skull and scalp. Look and feel for D-O-T-S. Check for clear fluid in ears (cerebrospinal fluid).

2. **Eyes:** Gently open both eyes and compare the pupils—they should be the same size. Check to see if they react to light.

3. **Neck:** Look and gently feel for D-O-T-S. Check for a medical-alert necklace.

4. **Chest:** Check for D-O-T-S. Gently squeeze the chest for rib pain.

5. **Abdomen:** Check for D-O-T-S. Gently press the four abdominal quadrants.

6. **Pelvis:** Check for D-O-T-S:
   a. Gently press downward on the tops of the hips for pain.
   b. Gently press towards each other for pain.

7. **Extremities:** Check the full length of both arms and legs for D-O-T-S. Check for CSM—circulation (pulse), sensation, movement.

Figure 1) D = Deformity

Figure 2) T = Tenderness

Figure 3) O = Open wounds

Figure 4) S = Swelling

abnormal shape.

Open wounds break the skin.

Tenderness is sensitivity to touch.

Swelling is the body's response to injury that makes the area look larger than usual

Here are some things you should look and feel for during the physical exam:

Head Have someone stabilize the victim's head and neck to keep it from moving. Look and feel for D-O-T-S over the entire head. Look for leakage of blood or fluid (cerebrospinal fluid) from the nose or ears.

Eyes Check the pupils of the eyes for equality and reactivity to light. Pupils should be of equal size when the brain is not injured. To check for reactivity to light, use a flashlight or cover and then uncover the victim's eyes with your hand. Pupils normally quickly constrict in response to light.

Neck Look and feel for D-O-T-S.

Chest Look and feel the entire chest for D-O-T-S. Squeeze or compress the sides together for rib pain.

Abdomen Look and feel for D-O-T-S. Gently press all

four abdominal quadrants for rigidity and tenderness, using the pads of your fingers. If the victim complains of pain in a particular area, ask the victim to point to it; press that area last.

Pelvis Look and feel for D-O-T-S. Gently squeeze the hips inward together and gently press the hips downward.

Extremities Look and feel the entire length and girth of each extremity (arms and legs) for D-O-T-S. Check the Circulation, Sensation, and Movement (use the mnemonic **CSM** as a way of remembering) of each extremity. Check for circulation in the arms by feeling for the radial pulse on the victim's thumb side of the wrist and check the circulation of the legs by feeling for the posterior tibial pulse between the inside of the ankle bone and the Achilles tendon. In a responsive victim, check for sensation by asking the victim whether he or she can feel you pinching his or her fingers and toes. To check for movement, ask the victim to wiggle his or her fingers and toes, to squeeze your hand with his or her hands, and to push his or her feet against your hand. Compare the responses of one extremity against the responses of the

C — CIRCULATION
S — SENSATION
M — MOVEMENT

CSM

other for any differences. Lack of sensation or movement can indicate an injured extremity or spinal injury.

If you suspect a spinal injury, do not move the victim's head or neck. Stabilize the victim against any movement, and be sure to tell him or her not to move.

SAMPLE History The information in a **SAMPLE** history can affect the first aid you give. It is called a SAMPLE history because the letters in the word "SAMPLE" stand for the elements of the history:

S = Symptoms

"What's wrong?" (known as the chief complaint)

A = Allergies

"Are you allergic to anything?"

M = Medications

"Are you taking any medications? What are they for?"

P = Past medical history

"Have you had this problem before? Do you have other medical problems?"

L = Last oral intake

"When did you last eat or drink anything? What was it?"

E = Events leading up to the illness or injury

Injury: "How did you get hurt?"
Illness: "What led to this problem?"

If the victim is unresponsive, you may be able to obtain the SAMPLE history information from family, friends, or bystanders.

Caution:

WHEN DOING A PHYSICAL EXAM

DO NOT aggravate injuries or contaminate wounds.

DO NOT move a victim with a possible spinal injury.

Physical Exam and SAMPLE History for Injured Victims

For an injured victim, start by reconsidering the cause (mechanism) of injury that you identified previously, during the scene survey (▶Table 1). This allows you to determine which procedures to use in checking an

---

Table 1: Significant Mechanisms (Causes) of Injury

- Falls of more than 15 feet for adults, more than 10 feet for children, or more than three times the victim's height

- Vehicle collisions involving ejection, a rollover, high speeds, a pedestrian, a motorcycle, or a bicycle

- Unresponsive or altered mental status

- Penetrations of the head, chest, or abdomen (eg, stab or gunshot wounds) of the muscle between the neck and shoulder

---

injured victim.

Injured Victim With a Significant Mechanism of Injury For an injured victim with a significant mechanism of injury, stabilize the head (if the injury involves the head, neck, chest, or back) to keep it from moving, check ABC, perform a rapid physical examination from head to toe, and if possible, obtain a SAMPLE history.

Injured Victim With No Significant Mechanism of Injury The physical examination of a victim without a significant mechanism of injury should focus on the area(s) that the victim complains about. Determine the chief complaint—the problem as the victim describes it. For example, the victim might complain of "twisting" an ankle. Begin the physical examination at the location of the injury using the mnemonic **D-O-T-S.** Your assessment focuses on just the areas that the victim tells you are painful or that you suspect may be injured. After the physical exam, conduct a SAMPLE history.

Physical Exam and SAMPLE History for Ill Victims

With a responsive ill victim, first obtain the victim's SAMPLE history then conduct a physical examination focused on the victim's chief complaint (symptoms). With an unresponsive ill victim, perform a rapid physical examination first, followed by the victim's SAMPLE history (if possible from bystanders).

Medical Identification Tags Look for medical identification tags, which may be beneficial in identifying allergies, medications, allergies, or medical history (▶Figure 5). A medical-alert tag, worn as a necklace or as a bracelet, contains the wearer's medical problem(s) and a 24-hour telephone number that offers, in case of an emergency, access to the victim's medical history plus names of doctors and close relatives. Necklaces and bracelets are durable, in-

Victim Assessment Sequence

Determine responsiveness

↓

Perform initial assessment (ABCs)

Injured Victim

1. Significant Mechanism of Injury:
   a. Physical exam (head to toe)
   b. SAMPLE history
2. No Significant Mechanism of Injury:
   a. Physical exam (examine only complaint)
   b. SAMPLE history

Ill Victim

1. Responsive:
   a. SAMPLE history
   b. Physical exam (examine only complaint)
2. Unresponsive:
   a. Physical exam (head to toe)
   b. SAMPLE history (from bystanders)

Figure 5 Medic Alert® identification tag

stantly recognizable, and less likely than cards to be separated from the victim in an emergency.

What to Do Until EMS Arrives

The initial assessment, physical examination, and SAMPLE history are done quickly so that injuries and illnesses can be identified and given first aid and, if necessary, transportation can be arranged. After the most serious problems have been cared for, regularly recheck the victim.

Recheck the victim's responsiveness, airway, breathing, circulation, and the effectiveness of first aid. Do this at least every 15 minutes for an alert victim, who has no serious injury or illness, and at least every five minutes for a victim who is unresponsive; has difficulties with airway, breathing, or circulation, including major blood loss; or has a significant mechanism of injury. Report your findings to EMS personnel when they arrive.

Meeting OSHA Guidelines

This chapter covers the following OSHA Guidelines for First Aid training:

- Section III. C. 1a-d. The assessment of scenes that require first aid services.
- Section III. C. 2. Performing a primary survey of each victim.
- Section III. C. 3. The techniques and principles of taking a victim's history at the scene of an emergency.
- Section III. C. 4. Performing a secondary survey of the victim.

Learning Activities

Finding Out What's Wrong

Directions: Circle Yes if you agree with the statement, and circle No if you disagree.

Yes No   1. The purpose of an initial assessment is to find life-threatening conditions.

Yes No   2. Crying or screaming victims should be treated before quiet ones.

Yes No   3. Most injured victims require a complete assessment.

Yes No   4. In a physical exam, you usually begin at the head and work down the body.

Yes No   5. Tapping a victim's shoulder helps in determining the victim's responsiveness.

Yes No   6. The mnemonic D-O-T-S helps in remembering what to collect about the victim's history that may be useful.

Yes No   7. For all injured and suddenly ill persons, look for medical-alert identification.

Yes No   8. The mnemonic SAMPLE can remind you how to examine an area for signs of an injury.

Scenario: During a mid-morning break, a coworker screams that somebody has collapsed in the hallway. As a company designated first aider, you push your way through a crowd of people gathered around the victim. You recognize Clyde, one of the older employees who is about to retire from the company, lying on the floor motionless. You notice that he wears a medical-alert identification bracelet.

_____9. After confirming that the scene is safe, you next check Clyde for:

     A. breathing   **B.** signs of circulation   **C.** broken bones   **D.** responsiveness

_____10. If he were unresponsive, you would:

     A. open his airway and check for breathing   **B.** look for signs of circulation
     C. look and feel for broken bones   **D.** look at his medical-alert ID tag

_____11. If Clyde were responsive and breathing, what would you next check?

     A. physical exam   **B.** victim's history

_____12. For injured victims, which usually comes first?

     A. physical exam   **B.** victim's history

_____13. The physical exam on an adult should be started at the victim's:

     A. head   **B.** chest   **C.** feet

_____14. Which of these would the medical-alert identification bracelet help identify?

     A. allergies   **B.** medications   **C.** medical history   **D.** all of these

_____15. When checking Clyde's eyes, you should look for:

     A. color of the iris   **B.** reaction of pupils to light
     C. equal or unequal size of the pupils   **D.** both B and C

Chapter 4

Basic Life Support

Heart attacks causing heart stoppage (cardiac arrest) are the most prominent cause of death in North America. In addition, drownings, suffocations, electrocutions, and drug intoxication cause cardiac arrest. Many deaths can be prevented if the victims receive early CPR, early automated external defibrillation (AED), and early advanced care by trained EMS professionals.

Rescue Breathing

For the breathing unresponsive victim, place him or her in the recovery position (▶ Figure 1). For the non-breathing victim, rescue breathing must be started immediately. Roll victim onto his or her back. If a victim is not breathing, perform rescue breathing by using one of the following methods: mouth-to-mouth, mouth-to-nose, mouth-to-stoma, or mouth-to-barrier device.

Mouth-to-Mouth Method

The mouth-to-mouth method of rescue breathing is a simple, quick, and effective method for an emergency situation. Pinch the victim's nose and breathe into the victim's mouth.

Mouth-to-Nose Method

Although mouth-to-mouth breathing is successful in the majority of cases, certain complications may necessitate mouth-to-nose rescue breathing; for example, if you cannot open the victim's mouth, their teeth are clenched together, you cannot make a good seal around the victim's mouth, the victim's mouth is severely injured, or the victim's mouth is too large or has no teeth.

The mouth-to-nose technique is performed like mouth-to-mouth breathing, except that you force your exhaled breath through the victim's nose while holding his or her mouth closed with one hand pushing up on the chin. The victim's mouth then must be held open so any nasal obstruction does not impede exhalation of air from the victim's lungs.

Figure 1 Recovery position. The hand supports the head. Head tilted. Bent knee and arm give stability.

Mouth-to-Stoma Method

Cancer and other diseases of the vocal cords often make surgical removal of the larynx necessary. People who have had this surgery breathe through a small permanent opening in the lower part of the neck called a *stoma*, which is surgically made and joined to the trachea.

In mouth-to-stoma rescue breathing, the victim's mouth and nose must be closed during the delivery of breaths because the air can flow upward into the upper airway through the larynx as well as downward into the lungs. You can close the victim's mouth and nose with one hand. Determine breathing by looking at, listening to, and feeling the stoma. Keep the victim's head and neck level.

Mouth-to-Barrier Device

A mouth-to-barrier device is an apparatus that is placed over a victim's face as a safety precaution for the rescuer during rescue breathing. There are two types of mouth-to-barrier devices:

- *Masks.* Resuscitation masks are clear, plastic devices that cover the victim's mouth and nose. They have a one-way valve so exhaled air from the victim does not enter the rescuer's mouth (▼Figure 2).
- *Face shields.* These clear plastic devices have a

Figure 2 Mouth-to-barrier device—mask.

Figure 3 Face shield

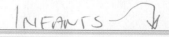

Gastric Distention

Rescue breathing can cause stomach or gastric distention more often in infants than in adults. Minimize this problem by limiting the breaths to the amount needed to make the chest rise. Avoid overinflating the lungs. Gastric distention can cause regurgitation and aspiration of stomach contents.

mouthpiece through which the rescuer breathes (▲Figure 3). Some models have a short airway that is inserted into the victim's mouth over the tongue. They are smaller and less expensive than masks, but air can leak around the shield. Also, they cover only the victim's mouth, so the nose must be pinched.

After the barrier device is in place, the rescuer breathes through the device. The technique is performed like mouth-to-mouth breathing. See the skill sheets in this chapter for the steps for performing rescue breathing.

Airway Obstruction (Choking)
Recognizing Choking

A foreign body lodged in the airway may cause partial or complete airway obstruction. When a foreign body partially blocks the airway, either good or poor air exchange may result. When good air exchange is present, the victim is able to make forceful coughing efforts in an attempt to relieve the obstruction. The victim should be permitted and encouraged to cough. Sometimes, however, a good air exchange may progress to a poor air exchange.

A choking victim who has poor air exchange has a weak and ineffective cough, and breathing becomes more difficult. The skin, the fingernail beds, and the inside of the

> ## Compression-Only CPR
> Some people are reluctant to perform mouth-to-mouth breathing on strangers for a variety of reasons, including fear of disease transmission. If a person is unwilling or unable to give mouth-to-mouth rescue breathing, chest compression-only CPR shoud be given rather than not trying at all.

> ## Defibrillation
> Most adults in cardiac arrest need to be defibrillated. Early defibrillation is the single most important factor in surviving cardiac arrest.
> See Appendix B for information on automated external defibrillators.

mouth may appear bluish-gray in color. Each attempt to inhale is usually accompanied by a high-pitched noise. A partial airway obstruction with poor air exchange should be treated as if it were a complete airway blockage.

Complete airway obstruction in a responsive victim commonly occurs when the victim has been eating. Children and infants choke on all kinds of objects. Foods such as hot dogs, candy, peanuts, and grapes are major offenders because of their shape and consistencies. Non-food choking deaths are caused by balloons, balls, marbles, toys, and coins. With complete airway obstruction, the victim is unable to speak, breathe, or cough. When asked, "Can you speak?" the victim is unable to respond verbally. Choking victims with complete foreign body obstruction of the airway may instinctively reach up and clutch their necks to communicate that they are choking. This motion is known as the distress signal for choking. The victim becomes panicked and desperate and may appear pale in color. Because a complete obstruction prevents air from entering the lungs, oxygen deprivation occurs within a few minutes.

Complete airway obstruction in an unresponsive victim is usually the result of the tongue relaxing in the back of the mouth, restricting air movement. Simple positioning of airway can correct this problem. See the skill sheets in this chapter for the steps for clearing an airway obstruction.

Cardiopulmonary Resuscitation (CPR)

One of the leading causes of death in the United States is sudden cardiac arrest, resulting in about 250,000 deaths each year.

Causes of Cardiac Arrest

Most sudden cardiac arrest victims have an electrical malfunction of the heart termed ventricular fibrillation. In ventricular fibrillation, the heart's electrical signals, which normally induce a coordinated heartbeat, suddenly become chaotic, and the heart's pumping function abruptly ceases. When the heart stops pumping blood, the

victim immediately loses consciousness and is considered clinically dead. A heart in ventricular fibrillation quivers like a bowl of gelatin. When this occurs, the heart is not pumping blood and there are only about four minutes to correct this problem before irreversible brain damage occurs. Without intervention, the victim will become biologically (irreversibly) dead within minutes. When a person's heart stops beating, he or she needs CPR. Refer to the Skill Sheets in this chapter for CPR procedures.

Infant Basic Life Support

Basic life support techniques for an infant differ from those for an adult or child. Initially occurring cardiac arrest in infants is rare. Usually, infants have a respiratory arrest with cardiac arrest developing later because the heart muscle did not receive sufficient oxygen.

Airway Obstruction—Infant

People, especially children and infants, inhale all kinds of objects. Foods such as hot dogs, candy, peanuts, and grapes are major offenders because of their shape and consistencies. Non-food choking deaths are caused by balloons, balls and marbles, toys, and coins.

As discussed before, the airway may be partially or completely blocked. With a partial airway obstruction, an infant is able to make persistent coughing efforts that should not be hampered. If good air exchange becomes a poor exchange or poor air exchange occurs initially, the victim should be managed as having a complete airway obstruction. Poor air exchanges are indicated by ineffective coughing, high-pitched noises, breathing difficulty, and blueness of the lips and fingernail beds.

> ### Meeting OSHA Guidelines
> This chapter covers the following OSHA Guidelines for First Aid training:
> - Section III. D. 1a-e. Basic Adult Cardiopulmonary Resuscitation (CPR) training.

BASIC LIFE SUPPORT

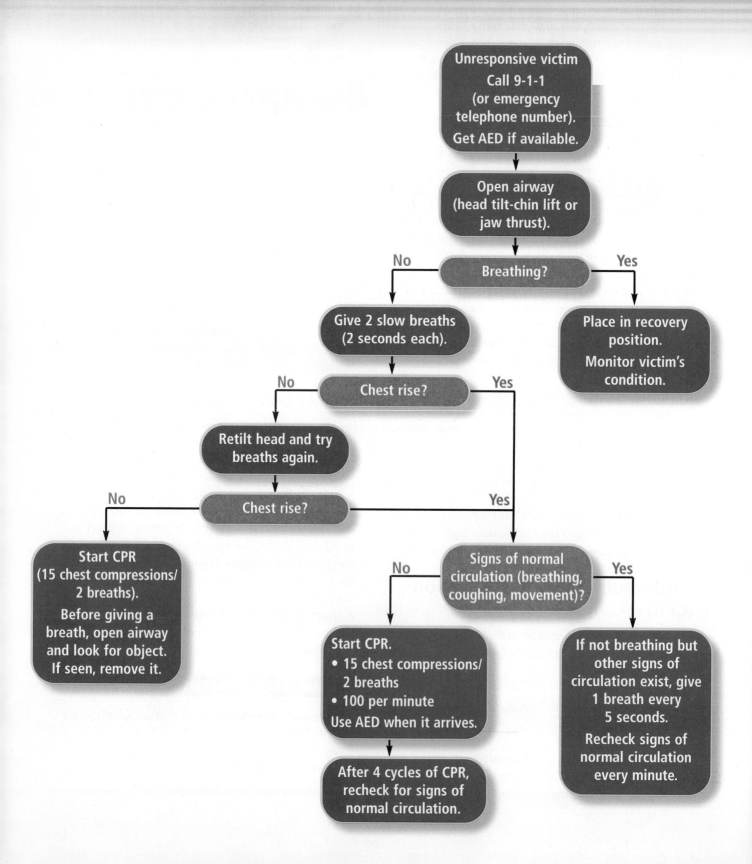

Basic Life Support
Adult and Child Rescue Breathing and CPR

If you see a motionless person ...

1

Check responsiveness.
- Tap victim and shout, "Are you okay?"
- If unresponsive, shout for help and go to step #2.

(speech bubble: Are you okay?)

2

Call 9-1-1 or emergency telephone number.
- If the victim is 8 years of age or older and an AED is available, get it.
- For an unresponsive child, continue assessment and resuscitation for 1 minute (if alone) and then call.

3

Open airway.
- Tilt the head back and lift the chin.
- Remove any obvious obstructions.
- If you suspect a spinal injury, use jaw-thrust method without head-tilt.

4

Check breathing (10 seconds).
- Look at the victim's chest for rise and fall; listen and feel for breathing.
- If breathing, place victim in recovery position.
- If not breathing, give 2 slow rescue breaths (2 seconds each).
- If breaths do not cause the chest to rise, the airway may be blocked. Reposition the head and try breaths again. If chest does not rise, begin CPR (see step #6). When you open the airway to give a breath, look for an object in the throat and if seen, remove it.
- If two breaths cause the chest to rise, continue to step #5.

Basic Life Support
Adult and Child Rescue Breathing and CPR

5

Check circulation (10 seconds).

Signs of circulation include—breathing, coughing, and movement (pulse checks can be done by healthcare providers).

If not breathing, but other signs of circulation exist, give one breath every 4–5 seconds. Recheck signs of circulation every minute.

If no signs of circulation exist, begin CPR (step #6).

6

Perform CPR.

• Place heel of one hand on the lower half of the sternum between the nipples.

• Using two hands, depress chest downward $1^1/_2$ to 2 inches.

• Give 15 chest compressions at a rate of about 100 per minute.

• Open airway and give two slow breaths (two seconds each).

• Continue cycles of 15 chest compressions and two rescue breaths.

• For a child (1 to 8), give chest compressions with 1 hand 5 times ($1–1^1/_2$ inches) followed by 1 breath.

Down-stroke Upstroke

Shoulders over hands

Straight arms

Pivot at hips

Use heel of hand

7

Recheck circulation.

After four cycles of compressions and breaths (about one minute), recheck for signs of circulation.

• If not breathing and no other signs of circulation exist, resume CPR.

Basic Life Support
Adult and Child Rescue Breathing and CPR

7 **continued**

- If breathing, place victim in recovery position.
- If not breathing, but other signs of circulation exist, provide one rescue breath about every five seconds.
- Recheck for signs of circulation every few minutes.

8

Early defibrillation

If you are trained to use an AED, follow this sequence:
- Perform CPR until an AED is available.
- Turn on the AED.
- Attach AED pads.
- "Analyze" the heart rhythm.
- Shock (up to three times if advised by AED).

After three shocks or after any AED prompt of "no shock indicated:"
- Check for signs of circulation (including carotid pulse).
- If no signs of circulation, perform CPR for one minute.

Check for signs of circulation. If absent:
- "Analyze" and continue to follow the AED's prompts.
- Shock, if prompted.
- Repeat, analyze, shock, and CPR as needed.

See Appendix B, Automated External Defibrillators (AEDs), for more detailed information about AED use.

Basic Life Support
Responsive Adult and Child Airway Obstruction

If person is responsive and cannot speak, breathe, or cough…

1

Check victim for choking.
- Ask "Are you choking? Can you speak?"
- A choking victim cannot speak, breathe or cough and may clutch the neck.

2

Give abdominal thrusts (Heimlich maneuver).
- Place a fist against the victim's abdomen just above the navel.
- Grasp the fist with your other hand and press into victim's abdomen with quick inward and upward thrusts.
- Continue thrusts until object is removed or victim becomes unresponsive.
- Give chest thrusts instead of abdominal thrusts for women in late stages of pregnancy or obese victims.

3

If the victim becomes unresponsive:
- Call 9-1-1 or emergency telephone number to activate the EMS system (or send someone to do it).
- Check victim and begin CPR.
- Each time you open the airway to give a breath, look for an object in the throat and if seen, remove it.

Basic Life Support
Infant Rescue Breathing and CPR

If you see a motionless infant …

1

Check responsiveness.

• Tap the victim and shout, "Are you okay?"

• If unresponsive, shout for help and go to step #2.

2

Call 9-1-1 or emergency telephone number.

• Ask a bystander to call.

• If you are alone, call 9-1-1 after one minute of resuscitation, unless a bystander can be sent. Infant may be carried to the telephone to call 9-1-1.

Open the airway.

• Tilt head back slightly and lift chin.

Check for breathing (10 seconds).

• Place your ear over the victim's mouth and nose while keeping the airway open.

• *Look* at the victim's chest for rise and fall; *listen* and *feel* for breathing.

If not breathing, give 2 slow breaths.

• Keep the airway open.

• Take a breath and place your mouth over the victim's mouth and nose, or nose only.

• Give 2 slow breaths (1–1$\frac{1}{2}$ seconds each)

• Watch chest rise to see if your breaths go in.

If breaths do not go in

Retilt the head and try again. If unsuccessful, the airway may be blocked. Begin CPR (step #7)

Basic Life Support
Infant Rescue Breathing and CPR

6

Check for signs of circulation (10 seconds).

Signs of circulation include breathing, coughing, and movement (pulse checks can be done by healthcare providers).

7

If not breathing, but other signs of circulation:

• Give 1 breath every 3 seconds.

• Recheck signs of circulation every minute (about 20 rescue breaths).

If there are no signs of circulation:

• Begin CPR.

   1. Place 2 fingers on the sternum about 1 finger width below imaginary nipple line.

   2. Compress the chest 5 times.

   3. Push sternum straight down $1/2$ to 1 inch ($1/3$ to $1/2$ depth of chest).

   4. Do smooth compressions, counting "One, two, three, four, five" (rate of 100 per minute).

• Give 1 slow breath.

• Continue cycles of 5 compressions and one breath for one minute (about 20 cycles), then check for signs of circulation. If absent, restart CPR with chest compressions. Recheck the signs of circulation every few minutes. If there are signs of circulation but no breathing, give rescue breathing.

• Give CPR until:

• Infant revives.

OR

• Trained help, such as emergency medical technicians (EMTs), arrives and relieves you.

OR

• You are completely exhausted.

Basic Life Support
Responsive Infant Airway Obstruction

If infant is responsive but cannot cry, breathe, or cough…

①

Give up to 5 back blows.
- Firmly support the infant's head and neck with 1 hand.
- Lay the infant face down over your forearm with head lower than his or her chest.
- Give up to 5 distinct and separate back blows between the infant's shoulder blades with the heel of your hand.

②

Give up to 5 chest thrusts.
- While supporting the back of the infant's head, roll the infant face up.
- Place your fingers on the infant's sternum.
- Give up to 5 separate and distinct thrusts with your index and middle fingers on the infant's sternum in same location used in CPR chest compressions.

③

Repeat.
- Until the infant becomes unresponsive. Call 9-1-1, assess infant and begin CPR if needed. Each time you open the airway to give a breath, look for an object in the throat and if seen, remove it.

OR

- Until object is expelled and infant begins to breathe or cough forcefully.

Basic Life Support Review

These techniques are the same for all victims regardless of age:

• Check responsiveness—tap and shout.
• Open airway—head tilt-chin lift; for suspected spinal injury use jaw-thrust without head tilt.
• Check breathing—look at chest to rise and fall and listen and feel for breathing.
• If breathing, place in recovery position.
• If not breathing, give 2 slow breaths (#1 in table).
• If breaths do not cause chest to rise, retilt head and give breaths again.
• If breaths still unsuccessful, give CPR (#2 in table).
• Check for signs of circulation (breathing, coughing, movement, normal skin condition).
• If not breathing but other signs of circulation exist, give rescue breaths (#3 in table).
• If not breathing and if no signs of circulation exist, give CPR (#4 in table).

Action	Adult (>8 years)	Child (1-8 years)	Infant (<1 year)
1. Breathing methods	Mouth-to-barrier device Mouth-to-mouth Mouth-to-nose Mouth-to-stoma	Mouth-to-barrier device Mouth-to-mouth Mouth-to-nose	Mouth-to-barrier device Mouth-to-mouth and nose Mouth-to-nose
2. Foreign-body airway obstruction in unresponsive victim	CPR cycles of 15 compressions to 2 breaths. Before giving a breath, look for an object in throat and if seen, remove it.	CPR cycles of 5 compressions to 1 breath. Before giving a breath, look for an object in throat and if seen, remove it.	CPR cycles of 5 compressions to 1 breath. Before giving a breath, look for an object in throat and if seen, remove it.
3. Rescue breathing	1 breath every 5 seconds. Should cause chest to rise.	1 breath every 3 seconds. Should cause chest to rise.	1 breath every 3 seconds. Should cause chest to rise.
4. Compressions:			
• Locating hand positions	• Lower half of sternum, between nipples	• Lower half of sternum, between nipples	• 1 finger width below nipple line
• Method	• Heel of 1 hand, other hand on top	• Heel of 1 hand	• 2 fingers
• Depth	• $1\frac{1}{2}$ inch to 2 inches	• 1 to $1\frac{1}{2}$ inches	• $\frac{1}{2}$ to 1 inch
• Rate	• 100 per minute	• 100 per minute	• 100+ per minute
• Ratio of chest compressions to breaths	• 15:2	• 5:1	• 5:1
5. When to activate EMS when alone	Immediately after establishing unresponsiveness	After 1 minute of resuscitation, unless bystander available who can call	After 1 minute of resuscitation, unless bystander available who can call
6. Automated external defibrillation (AED)	Yes	No	No

Learning Activities

Basic Life Support

Directions: Circle Yes if you agree with the statement; circle No if you disagree.

Yes (No) 1. Determine responsiveness by splashing cold water on the victim's face.

Yes (No) 2. Check for absent breathing by looking for widely dilated pupils.

(Yes) No 3. Take about 10 seconds when checking for breathing.

Yes (No) 4. If an adult victim is unresponsive, the first aider should call the local emergency telephone number immediately.

(Yes) No 5. Bending the head back and lifting the chin opens the airway.

(Yes) No 6. If you suspect a victim has a spinal injury, stabilize the head and lift the jaw.

Yes (No) 7. When checking for signs of circulation look for breathing, coughing, or movement.

(Yes) No 8. When giving chest compressions, push straight down on a victim's chest.

(Yes) No 9. Perform chest compressions with the victim on a level, firm surface.

(Yes) No 10. For adult and child CPR, give 5 compressions followed by 1 breath.

(Yes) No 11. Use two hands, one hand on top of the other, when performing CPR on an adult.

(Yes) No 12. One of the best signs of choking is that the victim is unable to speak or cough.

(Yes) No 13. To give abdominal thrusts to a responsive choking victim, place your fist below the victim's navel.

(Yes) No 14. Before giving a breath to an unresponsive choking victim, check the mouth for any obvious obstructions.

(Yes) No 15. When giving abdominal thrusts to a responsive choking victim, repeat until the object is removed or the victim becomes unresponsive.

(Yes) No 16. If the initial breaths did not go into an unresponsive choking victim, retilt the head and try more breaths.

(Yes) No 17. For an unresponsive choking adult, the rescuer should give CPR chest compressions.

Scenario #1: An older assembly line worker suddenly falls to the floor. She is unresponsive. What should you do?

_____

Scenario #2: A power company lineman is electrocuted and is unresponsive. What should you do?

_____

Scenario #3: A man in the company lunchroom surprises everyone around him by suddenly standing up and grabbing his throat. He is unable to speak and begins to turn blue. What should you do?

_____

Chapter 5

Bleeding and Shock

Bleeding

External Bleeding

External bleeding occurs when blood can be seen coming from an open wound. The term hemorrhage refers to a large amount of bleeding in a short time.

Types of External Bleeding

External bleeding can be classified into three types according to its source. In arterial bleeding, blood spurts (up to several feet) from the wound. Arterial bleeding is the most serious type of bleeding because blood is lost at a fast rate, leading to a large blood loss. Arterial bleeding also is less likely to clot because blood can clot only when it is flowing slowly or not at all. However, unless a very large artery has been cut, it is unlikely that a person will bleed to death before the flow can be controlled. Nevertheless, arterial bleeding is dangerous and must be controlled.

In venous bleeding, blood from a vein flows steadily or gushes. Venous bleeding is easier to control than arterial bleeding. Most veins collapse when cut. Bleeding from deep veins, however, can be as massive and as hard to control as arterial bleeding.

In capillary bleeding, the most common type of bleeding, blood oozes from capillaries. It usually is not serious and easily controlled. Often, this type of bleeding will clot and stop by itself.

What to Do

Regardless of the type of bleeding or the type of wound, the first aid is the same. First, and most important, you must control the bleeding (▶Skill Scan):

1. Protect yourself against disease by wearing medical exam gloves. If medical exam gloves are not available, use several layers of gauze pads, plastic wrap, a plastic bag, clean cloths or waterproof material.

Skill Scan   **Bleeding Control**

1a. Direct pressure stops most bleeding. Wear medical exam gloves, and place a sterile gauze pad or a clean cloth over wound.

1b. A pressure bandage can free you to attend to other injuries or victims.

2. If bleeding continues, use elevation to help reduce blood flow. Combine with direct pressure over the wound.

3. If bleeding continues, apply pressure at a pressure point to slow blood flow. Locations are:

(**a**) brachial or (**b**) femoral. Combine with direct pressure over the wound.

You can even have the victim apply pressure on the wound with his or her own hand. After bleeding has stopped and the wound has been cared for, vigorously wash your hands with soap and water.

2. Expose the wound by removing or cutting the clothing to find the source of the blood.

Caution:

DO NOT touch a wound with your bare hands. If you must use your bare hands, do so only as a last resort. After the bleeding has stopped and the wound has been cared for, vigorously wash your hands with soap and water.

DO NOT use direct pressure on an eye injury, a wound with an embedded object, or a skull fracture.

DO NOT remove a blood-soaked dressing. Apply another dressing on top and keep pressing.

3. Place a sterile gauze pad or a clean cloth such as a handkerchief, washcloth, or towel over the entire wound and apply direct pressure with your fingers or the palm of your hand. Hold steady, firm pressure uninterrupted for at least 5 minutes.

4. If bleeding is from an arm or leg, elevate the injured area above heart level as you continue to apply pressure to reduce blood flow. Elevating the extremity means that gravity will make it difficult for the body to pump blood to the affected limb.

5. If the bleeding continues, keep applying direct pressure over the wound and apply pressure at a pressure point to slow the flow of blood. A pressure point is where an artery near the skin's surface passes close to a bone, against which it can be compressed. The most accessible pressure points on both sides of the body are the brachial point in the upper inside arm and the femoral point in the groin.

6. To free you to attend to other injuries or victims, use a pressure bandage to hold the dressing on the wound. Wrap a roller gauze bandage tightly over the dressing and above and below the wound site.

7. When you cannot apply direct pressure (eg, in the case of a protruding bone, skull fracture, or embedded object), use a doughnut-shaped (ring) pad to control bleeding. (See Chapter 9, Head and Spinal Injuries.) To make a ring pad, wrap one end of a narrow bandage (roller or cravat) several times around your four fingers to form a loop. Pass the other end of the bandage through the loop and wrap it around and around until the entire bandage is used and a ring has been made.

8. When bleeding stops, use procedures in Chapter 6 for wound care.

Caution:

Tourniquets are rarely needed and can damage nerves and blood vessels. Using a tourniquet may cause the loss of an arm or leg. If you do use one, apply wide, flat materials—never rope or wire—and do not loosen it.

Internal Bleeding

Internal bleeding occurs when the skin is not broken and blood is not seen. It can be difficult to detect but can be life threatening. Internal bleeding comes from injuries that do not break the skin or from nontraumatic disorders such as ulcers.

What to Look For

The signs of internal bleeding may take days to appear:

- bruises or contusions of the skin
- painful, tender, rigid, bruised abdomen
- vomiting or coughing up blood
- stools that are black or contain bright red blood

What to Do

For severe internal bleeding, follow these steps:

1. Monitor ABCs.

2. Expect vomiting. If vomiting occurs, keep the victim lying on his or her left side for so that the vomiting can drain. This will also prevent the victim from inhaling vomitus and will prevent expulsion of vomit from the stomach.

3. Treat for shock by raising the victim's legs 8 to 12 inches and covering the victim with a coat or blanket to keep him or her warm. See page 38 for when to use other body positions.

4. Seek immediate medical attention.

Bruises are a form of internal bleeding but are not life threatening. To treat bruises see page 89.

BLEEDING

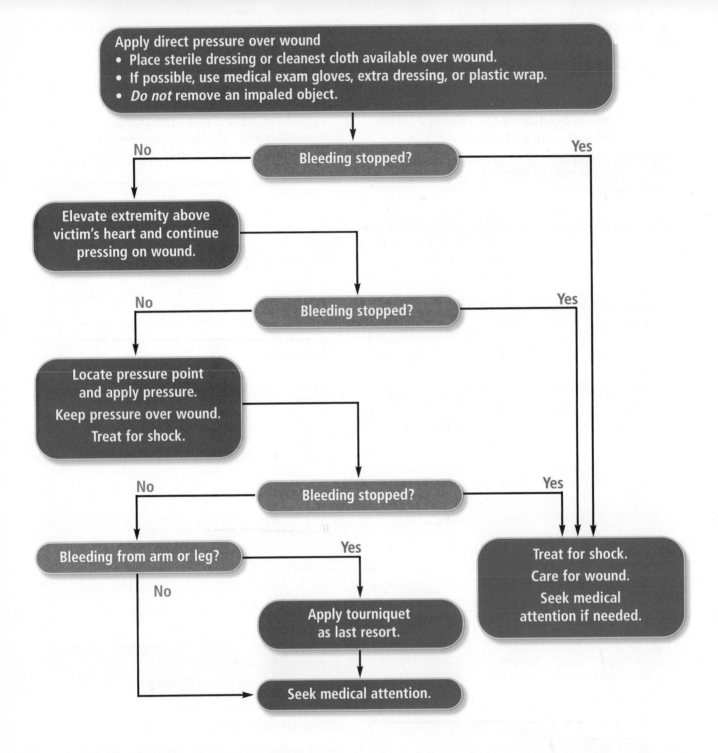

Apply direct pressure over wound
- Place sterile dressing or cleanest cloth available over wound.
- If possible, use medical exam gloves, extra dressing, or plastic wrap.
- *Do not* remove an impaled object.

No ← Bleeding stopped? → Yes

Elevate extremity above victim's heart and continue pressing on wound.

No ← Bleeding stopped? → Yes

Locate pressure point and apply pressure.
Keep pressure over wound.
Treat for shock.

No ← Bleeding stopped? → Yes

Bleeding from arm or leg? → Yes

No

Apply tourniquet as last resort.

Treat for shock.
Care for wound.
Seek medical attention if needed.

Seek medical attention.

Caution:

DO NOT give a victim anything to eat or drink. It could cause nausea and vomiting, which could result in inhaling foreign material into the lungs (aspiration). Food or liquids could cause complications during surgery if it is needed.

Shock

Shock refers to circulatory system failure, which happens when insufficient amounts of oxygenated blood is provided for every body part. Because every injury affects the circulatory system to some degree, first aiders should automatically treat injured victims for shock.

To understand shock, think of the circulatory system as having three components: a working pump (the heart), a network of pipes (the blood vessels), and an adequate amount of fluid (the blood) pumped through the pipes. Damage to any of these components can deprive tissues of blood and produce the condition known as shock.

Shock can be classified as one of three types according to which component fails.

- *Pump failure:* the heart cannot pump sufficient blood. For example, a major heart attack can damage the heart muscle so the heart cannot squeeze and therefore cannot push blood through the blood vessels.
- *Fluid loss:* a significant amount of fluid, usually blood, is lost from the system.
- *Pipe failure:* blood vessels (pipes) enlarge and the blood supply is insufficient to fill them. This can result when the nervous system is damaged, such as with a spinal injury or drug overdose).

What to Look For

- altered mental status: anxiety and restlessness
- pale, cold, and clammy skin, lips, and nail beds
- nausea and vomiting
- rapid breathing and pulse
- unresponsiveness when shock is severe

What to Do

Even if an injured victim does not have signs or symptoms of shock, first aiders should treat for shock ▶ Skill Scan .

1. Treat life-threatening injuries and other severe injuries.
2. Lay the victim on his or her back.
3. Raise the victim's legs 8 to 12 inches. Raising the legs allows the blood to drain from the legs back to the heart ▶ Skill Scan .
4. Prevent body heat loss by putting blankets and coats under and over the victim.

Anaphylaxis

A powerful reaction to substances eaten or injected can occur within minutes or even seconds. This reaction, called **anaphylaxis,** can cause death if it is not treated immediately.

Common Causes of Anaphylaxis

Well-known causes of anaphylaxis include:

- medications (penicillin and related drugs, aspirin, sulfa drugs)
- food and food additives (shellfish, nuts, eggs, monosodium glutamate, nitrates, nitrites)
- insect stings (honeybee, yellow jacket, wasp, hornet, fire ant)
- plant pollen
- radiographic dyes

Caution:

DO NOT mistake anaphylaxis for other reactions such as hyperventilation, anxiety attacks, alcohol intoxication, or low blood sugar.

What to Look For

Anaphylaxis typically comes on within minutes of exposure to the offending substance, peaks in 15 to 30 minutes, and is over within hours.

Signs and symptoms of anaphylaxis include:

- sneezing, coughing, wheezing
- shortness of breath
- tightness and swelling in the throat
- tightness in the chest

Skill Scan

Positioning the Shock Victim

1. Usual shock position. Elevate the legs 8 to 12 inches (if spinal injury is not suspected).

2. Elevate the head for head injury (if spinal injury not suspected).

3. Lay an unresponsive, breathing victim on his or her side.

4. Use a half-sitting position for those with breathing difficulties, chest injuries, or a heart attack.

5. Keep victim flat if a spinal injury is suspected or victim has leg fractures.

Figure 1 A–B **A.** Doctor-prescribed preloaded epinephrine autoinjector. **B.** Doctor-prescribed preloaded epinephrine with 2 shots.

- increased pulse rate
- swelling of the mucous membranes (tongue, mouth, nose)
- blueness around lips and mouth
- dizziness
- nausea and vomiting

What to Do

1. Check ABCs.
2. Seek immediate medical attention.
3. If the victim has his or her own physician-prescribed epinephrine, help the victim use it (◄ Figure 1 A–B).

Meeting OSHA Guidelines

This chapter covers the following OSHA Guidelines for First Aid training:

- Section IV. A. 1a-b. Instructions in the principles and first aid intervention in shock due to injury and allergic reactions.
- Section IV. A. 2a-b. The types of bleeding and the principles and performance of bleeding control interventions.

Learning Activities

Bleeding

Directions: Circle Yes if you agree with the statement, and circle No if you disagree.

Yes (No) 1. Most cases of bleeding require more than direct pressure to stop the bleeding.

Yes (No) 2. Remove and replace blood-soaked dressings.

(Yes) No 3. Elevating an arm or leg alone will not control bleeding and must be used in combination with direct pressure over the wound.

Yes (No) 4. If direct pressure and elevation fail to control bleeding, the next step would be to use a tourniquet.

(Yes) No 5. Applying pressure to pressure points in the arms or legs is often needed to control bleeding.

Scenario: Jim, a 25-year-old construction worker, has been badly cut on his thigh by a circular power saw. Blood is flowing heavily. The cut is about six to eight inches long. What should you do?

_____

_____

_____

_____

Shock

Yes (No) 1. Most victims of shock should be placed flat on their backs.

Yes (No) 2. Give the victim something to drink.

(Yes) No 3. Prevent body heat loss by putting blankets under and over the victim.

Yes (No) 4. A shock victim with head injuries should be placed on his or her side.

Yes (No) 5. A shock victim with breathing difficulty or chest injury should be placed on his or her back with the legs raised.

Scenario: You have controlled the construction worker's bleeding. He appears to be pale and is anxious and restless. What should you do?

_____

_____

_____

Anaphylaxis

Yes (No) 1. Anaphylaxis is another form of fainting.

(Yes) No 2. Anaphylaxis can kill.

(Yes) No 3. Ask the victim if he or she has a doctor-prescribed epinephrine injector.

Scenario: On a nice summer day, Susan is weeding in the front of the company's office building. Suddenly, she begins slapping her legs. She has disturbed a nest of yellow jackets, and is stung more than a dozen times. Susan complains that she feels hot, and has begun coughing, sneezing, and wheezing. You notice that her face seems to be getting puffy. What should you do?

_____

_____

_____

Chapter 6

Wounds

Open Wounds

An open wound is a break in the skin's surface that results in external bleeding and may allow bacteria to enter the body, causing infection.

There are several types of open wounds. Recognizing the type of wound helps in giving proper first aid. With an **abrasion** (▶Figure 1A), the top layer of skin is removed, with little or no blood loss. Abrasions tend to be painful, because the nerve endings often are torn along with the skin. Ground-in debris may be present. This type of wound can be serious if it covers a large area or becomes embedded with foreign matter. Other names for an abrasion are "scrape," "road rash," and "rug burn."

A **laceration** (▶Figure 1B) is cut skin with jagged, irregular edges. This type of wound is usually caused by a forceful tearing away of skin tissue.

Incisions (▶Figure 1C) tend to have smooth edges and resemble a surgical or paper cut. The amount of bleeding depends on the depth, the location, and the size of the wound.

Punctures (▶Figure 1D) are usually deep, narrow wounds such as a stab wound from a nail or a knife in the skin and underlying organs. The entrance is usually small, and the risk of infection is high. The object causing the injury may remain impaled in the wound.

With an **avulsion** (▶Figure 1E), a piece of skin is torn loose and is either hanging from the body or completely removed. This type of wound can bleed heavily. If the flap is still attached and folded back, lay it flat and align it in its normal position. Avulsions most often involve ears, fingers, and hands.

An **amputation** involves the cutting or tearing off of a body part, such as a finger, toe, hand, foot, arm, or leg.

What to Do

1. Protect yourself against disease by wearing medical exam gloves. If medical exam gloves are not available, use several layers of gauze pads, clean cloths, plastic wrap or bags, or waterproof material. You

Figure 1A Abrasion

Figure 1B Laceration

Figure 1C Incision

Figure 1D Puncture

Figure 1E Avulsion

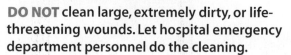

Caution:

DO NOT clean large, extremely dirty, or life-threatening wounds. Let hospital emergency department personnel do the cleaning.

DO NOT scrub a wound. Scrubbing a wound is debatable, and it can bruise the tissue.

Wound Care

A victim's wound should be cleaned to help prevent infection. Wound cleaning usually restarts bleeding by disturbing the clot, but it should be done anyway for shallow wounds. For severe bleeding, leave the pressure bandage in place until the victim can get medical attention. To clean a shallow wound:

1. Wash inside the wound with soap and water.

2. Irrigate the wound with water from a faucet to provide sufficient quantity and pressure.

can even have the victim apply pressure with his or her own hand. Your bare hand should be used only as a last resort.

2. Expose the wound by removing or cutting clothing to see where the blood is coming from.

3. Control bleeding as described in Chapter 5.

For a wound with a high risk for infection (eg, an animal bite, a very dirty or ragged wound, a puncture), seek medical attention for wound cleaning.

3. Remove small objects that don't flush out by irrigation with sterile tweezers.

4. If bleeding restarts, apply direct pressure.

5. Apply an antibiotic ointment such as Neosporin™. Cover the area with a sterile and, if possible, nonstick dressing. To keep the dressing in place on an arm or leg, use a self-adhering roller bandage or tape; on other parts of the body, use tape.

6. Change the dressing daily, or more often if it gets wet or dirty. If a wound bleeds after a dressing has been applied and the dressing becomes stuck, leave it on as long as the wound is healing. Pulling the scab loose to change the dressing retards healing and increases the chance of infection. If a sticking dressing must be removed, soak it in warm water to help soften the scab and make removal easier.

Caution:

DO NOT irrigate a wound with full-strength iodine preparations (eg, Betadine 10%) or isopropyl alcohol (70%). They kill body cells as well as bacteria and are painful. Also, some people are allergic to iodine.

DO NOT use hydrogen peroxide. It does not kill bacteria, it adversely affects capillary blood flow, and it extends wound healing.

DO NOT use antibiotic ointment on wounds that require sutures or on puncture wounds (the ointment may prevent drainage). Use an antibiotic ointment only on abrasions and shallow wounds.

Wound Infection

Any wound, large or small, can become infected . Once an infection begins, damage can be extensive, so prevention is the best way to avoid the problem. A wound should be cleaned using the procedures described above.

It is important to know how to recognize and treat an infected wound. The signs and symptoms of infection include:

Figure 2   Infected wound

- swelling and redness around the wound
- a sensation of warmth
- throbbing pain
- pus discharge
- fever
- swelling of lymph nodes
- one or more red streaks leading from the wound toward the heart

The appearance of one or more red streaks leading from the wound toward the heart is a serious sign that the infection is spreading and could cause death. If chills and fever develop, the infection has reached the circulatory system (known as blood poisoning). Seek medical attention immediately.

Tetanus

The tetanus bacteria by itself does not cause tetanus. But when it enters a wound that contains little oxygen (eg, a puncture wound), the bacteria can produce a powerful poisonous toxin. The toxin travels through the nervous system to the brain and the spinal cord. It then causes contractions of certain muscle groups (particularly in the jaw). There is no known antidote to the toxin after it enters the nervous system.

A vaccination can completely prevent tetanus. Everyone needs an initial series of vaccinations to prepare the immune system to defend against the toxin. A booster shot once every 5 to 10 years is sufficient to jog the immune system's memory.

The guidelines for tetanus immunization boosters are as follows:

- Anyone with a wound who has never been immunized against tetanus should be given a tetanus vaccine and booster immediately.

- A victim who was once immunized but has not received a tetanus booster within the last 10 years should receive a booster.

- A victim with a dirty wound who has not had a booster for over five years should receive a booster.

- Tetanus immunization shots must be given within 72 hours of the injury to be effective.

Amputations ▼Figure 3

What to Do

1. Control the bleeding.

2. Treat the victim for shock.

3. Recover the amputated part and, whenever possible, take it with the victim.

4. To care for the amputated body part ▶Figure 4 :

    - The amputated part does not need to be cleaned.

    - Wrap the amputated part with a dry sterile gauze or other clean cloth.

    - Put the wrapped amputated part in a plastic bag or other waterproof container.

    - Keep the amputated part cool, but do not freeze. Place the bag or container with the wrapped part on a bed of ice.

5. Seek medical attention immediately.

Amputated body parts left uncooled for more than six hours have little chance of survival; 18 hours is probably the maximum time allowable for a part that has been cooled properly. Muscles without blood lose viability within four to six hours.

Figure 3 Amputation

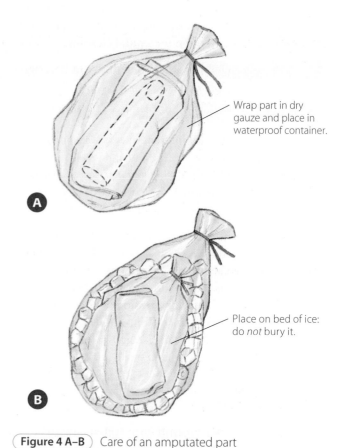

Wrap part in dry gauze and place in waterproof container.

A

Place on bed of ice: do *not* bury it.

B

Figure 4 A–B Care of an amputated part

Caution:

DO NOT wrap an amputated part in a wet dressing or cloth. Using a wet wrap on the part can cause waterlogging and tissue softening, which will make reattachment more difficult.

DO NOT bury an amputated part in ice—place it on ice. Reattaching frostbitten parts is usually unsuccessful.

Impaled Objects

What to Do

1. Expose the area ▶Figure 5 . Remove or cut away clothing surrounding the injury.

2. Do not remove or move an impaled object. Movement of any kind could produce additional bleeding and tissue damage.

3. Control any bleeding with pressure around the impaled object.

Figure 5 Impaled object

4. Stabilize the object with bulky dressings or clean cloths around the object.

5. Shorten the object only if necessary.

Closed Wounds

A closed wound happens when a blunt object strikes the body. The skin is not broken, but tissue and blood vessels beneath the skin's surface are crushed, causing bleeding within a confined area.

What to Do

1. Control bleeding by applying an ice pack for up to 20 minutes.

2. Apply an elastic bandage with a gauze pad between the bandage and the skin.

3. Check for a possible fracture.

4. Elevate an injured extremity above the victim's heart level to decrease pain and swelling.

Wounds That Require Medical Attention

As a guideline, seek medical attention for the following conditions:

- arterial bleeding
- uncontrolled bleeding
- a deep incision, laceration, or avulsion that
  - goes into the muscle or bone

- is located on a body part that bends such as the elbow or knee
  - tends to gape widely
  - is located on the thumb or palm of the hand (nerves may be affected)
- a large or deep puncture wound
- a large embedded object or a deeply embedded object of any size
- foreign matter left in the wound
- human or animal bite
- possibility of a noticeable scar (sutured cuts usually heal with less scarring than unsutured ones)
- an eyelid cut (to prevent later drooping)
- a slit lip (easily scarred)
- internal bleeding
- any wound you are not certain how to treat
- tetanus immunization not up to date

Sutures (Stitches)

If sutures are needed, they should be made by a physician within six to eight hours of the injury. Suturing wounds allows faster healing, reduces infection, and lessens scarring.

Some wounds do not usually require sutures:

- wounds in which the skin's cut edges tend to fall together
- shallow cuts less than one inch long

Rather than close a gaping wound with butterfly bandages, cover the wound with sterile gauze. Closing the wound might trap bacteria inside, resulting in an infection. In most cases, a physician can be reached in time for sutures to be made.

Meeting OSHA Guidelines

This chapter covers the following OSHA Guidelines for First Aid training:

- Section IV. A. 2c. The assessment and approach to wounds including abrasions, incisions, lacerations, punctures, avulsions, amputations, and crash injuries.

- Section IV. A. 2d. The principles of wound care including infection precautions, wounds requiring medical attention, and the need for tetanus prophylaxis.

- Section IV. A. 7b. Appropriate handling of amputated fingers, hands, and feet during the immediate transportation of the victim and body part to the hospital.

Learning Activities

Wound Care

Directions: Circle Yes if you agree with the statement, and circle No if you disagree.

(Yes) No   **1.** Wash shallow wounds with soapy water.

(Yes) No   **2.** Irrigating a wound with water needs pressure.

(Yes) No   **3.** Wounds with a high risk for infection (eg, animal bites, dirty wounds) require medical attention for proper wound cleaning.

Yes (No)   **4.** Antibiotic ointment can be applied to any wound.

Yes (No)   **5.** Hydrogen peroxide works well on wounds.

Scenario: Nancy used a knife to open a cardboard box, lost her grip on the knife, and received a shallow incision wound on her hand. What should you do?

_____

_____

_____

Amputations

(Yes) No   **1.** Recover any amputated part, regardless of size, and take it with the victim to the nearest hospital.

Yes (No)   **2.** Cut off a partially attached part.

(Yes) No   **3.** Wrap an amputated part in a dry, sterile gauze dressing, enclose it in something waterproof, and keep it cool.

Yes (No)   **4.** Keep an amputated part packed (buried) in ice.

(Yes) No   **5.** Do **NOT** let an amputated part become "water-logged" because reattaching it will be more difficult.

Scenario: Matt is mowing long wet grass, which begins to clog his mower's discharge opening. He reaches into the discharge chute to try to pull out the grass, and his fingers are struck by the mower's blade. Two fingers are cut off. You find him sitting on the ground firmly holding what remains of his fingers. What should you do?

_____

_____

_____

Impaled Objects

(Yes) No   **1.** Removing an impaled object could cause more bleeding.

(Yes) No   **2.** Prevent an impaled object from moving by placing bulky padding around the object.

Scenario: At a construction site, a worker drove a large nail through his left hand with a nail gun. What should you do?

_____

_____

_____

Chapter 7

Dressings and Bandages

Dressings

A dressing covers an open wound—it touches the wound. Whenever possible, a dressing should be:

- sterile. If a sterile dressing is not available, use a clean cloth (handkerchief, washcloth, towel).
- larger than the wound
- thick, soft, and compressible so pressure is evenly distributed over the wound
- lint-free

The purpose of a dressing is to:

- control bleeding
- prevent infection and contamination
- absorb blood and fluid drainage
- protect the wound from further injury

Types of Dressings

- *Gauze pads* are used for small wounds (▶Figure 1). They come in separately wrapped packages of various sizes (eg, 2 inches square; 4 inches square) and are sterile, unless the package is broken. Some gauze pads have a special coating to keep them from sticking to the wound and are especially helpful for burns or wounds secreting fluids.
- *Adhesive strips* (eg, Band-Aids™) are used for small cuts and abrasions and are a combination of both a sterile dressing and a bandage (▶Figure 2).
- *Trauma dressings* are made of large, thick, absorbent, sterile materials (▶Figure 3). Individually wrapped sanitary napkins can serve because of their bulk and absorbency, but they usually are not sterile.

Applying a Sterile Dressing
What to Do

1. Wear medical exam gloves whenever possible.
2. Use a dressing large enough to extend beyond the wound's edges. Hold the dressing by a corner. Place

the dressing directly over the wound. Do not slide it on.

3. Cover the dressing with one of the types of bandages referenced below.

Figure 1 Gauze pads

Figure 2 Adhesive strips

Figure 3 Trauma dressings

Caution:

DO NOT touch any part of the wound or any part of the dressings that will be in contact with the wound.

Bandages

A bandage can be used to:

- hold a dressing in place over an open wound
- apply direct pressure over a dressing to control bleeding
- prevent or reduce swelling
- provide support and stability for an extremity or joint

A bandage should be clean but need not be sterile.

Caution:

DO NOT bandage so tightly as to restrict blood circulation. Always check the extremity's pulse. If you cannot feel the pulse, loosen the bandage.

DO NOT bandage so loosely that the dressing will slip. This is the most common bandaging error. Bandages tend to stretch after a short time.

DO NOT cover fingers or toes unless they are injured. They need to be observed for color changes due to impaired circulation.

DO NOT use elastic bandages over a wound. First aiders have a tendency to apply them too tightly.

Signs that a bandage is too tight:

- blue tinge to the fingernails or toenails
- blue or pale skin color
- tingling or loss of sensation
- coldness of the extremity
- inability to move the fingers or toes

Types of Bandages

There are four basic types of bandages:

- **Roller bandages** come in various widths, lengths, and types of material. For best results, use different widths for different body areas (▶ **Skill Scans**):

- 1-inch width for fingers
- 2-inch width for wrists, hands, feet
- 3-inch width for elbows, arms
- 4- or 6-inch width for ankles, knees, legs

These can be *self-adhering, conforming bandages* (▼Figure 4) that come as rolls of slightly elastic, gauzelike material in various widths. They can also be g*auze rollers* made of cotton. These are rigid and nonelastic. Another type of roller bandage is an e*lastic roller bandage* used for compression on sprains, strains, and contusions. Elastic bandages are not usually applied over dressings to cover a wound.

When commercial roller bandages are unavailable, you can *improvise bandages* from neckties or strips of cloth torn from a sheet or other similar material.

- ***Triangular bandages*** (▶Figure 5) are available commercially or can be made from a 36- to 40-inch square of preshrunk cotton muslin material that is cut diagonally from corner to corner to produce two triangular pieces of cloth. The longest side is called the ***base***; the corner directly across from the base is the ***point***; the other two corners are called ***ends***. A triangular bandage may be applied two ways:

  - As a cravat (folded triangular bandage). The point is folded to the center of the base and folded in half again from the top to the base

Figure 5 A triangular bandage folded into a cravat

to form a cravat. It is to apply pressure evenly over a dressing, to hold splints in place, or used as a swathe (binder) around the victim's body to stabilize an injured arm in an arm sling.

  - Fully opened (not folded). Best used for an arm sling.

- ***Adhesive tape*** comes in rolls and in a variety of widths. It is often used to secure roller bandages and small dressings in place. Paper tape or special dermatologic tape should be used if the victim has an allergy to adhesive tape.

- ***Adhesive strips*** are used for small cuts and abrasions and are a combination of a dressing and a bandage.

Meeting OSHA Guidelines

This chapter covers the following OSHA Guidelines for First Aid training:

- Section IV. E. 1. Principles and performance of bandaging the head, chest, shoulder, arm, leg, wrist, elbow, foot, ankle, finders, toes, and knee.

Figure 4 Self-adhering conforming bandages of various sizes (3 on right) and gauze bandages (2 on left)

Skill Scan   Roller Bandage

Roller Bandage for Hand

1. Anchor the bandage with one or two turns around the palm of the hand.

2. Carry it diagonally across the back of the hand and then around the wrist.

3. Repeat this figure-8 maneuver with overlapping wraps.

Roller Bandage for Elbow or Knee

1. Bend arm. Wrap the bandage around the elbow several times.

2. Make a diagonal turn to the upper arm.

3. Make a diagonal turn around the forearm and continue this figure-8 maneuver.

Skill Scan

Roller Bandage (Self-adhering), Figure 8

Roller Bandage for Ankle

1. Anchor the bandage with one or two turns around the foot. Bring bandage diagonally across the top of the foot and around back of the ankle.

2. Continue bandage across the top of the foot and under the arch.

3. Continue figure-8 turns, with each turn overlapping the last turn.

Learning Activities

Dressings and Bandages

Directions: Circle Yes if you agree with the statement, and circle No if you disagree.

Yes   No   **1.** Bandages are used to secure dressings in place over a wound.

Yes   No   **2.** Dressings are used to control bleeding and prevent contamination.

Yes   No   **3.** Adhesive strips are types of bandages used for large wounds.

Yes   No   **4.** Fingers and toes should not be covered unless they are injured.

Yes   No   **5.** Triangular bandages can be used to control bleeding or to support splints for broken bones.

Scenario: A child "skinned" his knee when he fell off his bike. What should you do for this child?

_____

_____

_____

_____

Scenario: A worker has cut the palm of his hand on a sharp piece of metal. What should you do?

_____

_____

_____

_____

Chapter 8

Burns

Burn injuries can be classified as thermal (heat), chemical, or electrical.

- *Thermal (heat) burns.* Not all thermal burns are caused by flames. Contact with hot objects, flammable vapor that ignites and causes a flash or an explosion, and steam or hot liquid are other common causes of burns.

- *Chemical burns.* A wide range of chemical agents can cause tissue damage and death if they come in contact with the skin. As with thermal burns, the amount of tissue damage depends on the duration of contact, the skin thickness in the area of exposure, and the strength of the chemical agent. Chemicals will continue to cause tissue destruction until the chemical agent is removed. Three types of chemicals—acids, alkalis, and organic compounds—are responsible for most chemical burns.

- *Electrical burns.* The severity of an injury from contact with electrical current depends on the type of current (direct or alternating), the voltage, the area of the body exposed, and the duration of contact.

Historically, burns have been described as *first-degree*, *second-degree*, and *third-degree* injuries. The terms *superficial*, *partial thickness*, and *full thickness* are often used by burn-care professionals because they are more descriptive of the tissue damage.

- **First-degree (superficial) burns** affect the skin's outer layer (epidermis) ⟨ ▶Figure 1 ⟩. Characteristics include redness, mild swelling, tenderness, and pain. Healing occurs without scarring, usually within a week. The outer edges of deeper burns often are first-degree burns.

- **Second-degree (partial-thickness) burns** extend through the entire outer layer and into the inner skin layer ⟨ ▶Figure 2 ⟩. Blisters, swelling, weeping of fluids, and severe pain characterize these burns, because the capillary blood vessels in the dermis are damaged and give up fluid into surrounding tissues. Intact blisters provide a sterile, waterproof covering.

Figure 1   First-degree burn

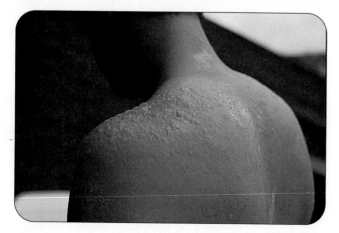

Figure 2   Second-degree burn blisters

Once a blister breaks, a weeping wound results and the risk of infection increases.

- **Third-degree (full-thickness) burns** are severe burns that penetrate all the skin layers, into the underlying fat and muscle (▶Figure 3). The skin looks leathery, waxy, or pearly gray and sometimes charred. There is a dry appearance, because capillary blood vessels have been destroyed and no more fluid is brought to the area. The skin does not blanch after being pressed because the area is dead. The victim feels no pain from a third-degree burn because the nerve endings have been damaged or destroyed. Any pain that is felt is from surrounding burns of lesser degrees. Medical care for a third-degree burn involves removing the dead tissue and often a skin graft to heal properly.

Respiratory damage may result from breathing heat or the products of combustion; from being burned by a

Figure 3   Second- and third-degree burns

flame while in a closed space; or from being in an explosion. Swelling occurs in 2 to 24 hours, restricting or even completely shutting off the airway so that air cannot reach the lungs. *All respiratory injuries must receive medical care.*

Thermal Burns
What to Do

1. Stop the burning! Burns can continue to injure tissue for a surprisingly long time. If clothing is burning, have the victim roll on the ground using the "stop, drop, and roll" method. Smother the flames with a blanket or douse the victim with water. Stop a person whose clothes are on fire from running, which only fans the flames. The victim should not remain standing, because he or she is more apt to inhale flames.

2. Check ABC.

3. Determine the depth (degree) of the burn. Making an assessment of burn depth will help you decide whether to seek medical care for the victim. You should be aware that it can be difficult to tell a burn's depth because the destruction varies within the same burn. Even experienced physicians may not know the true depth for several days after the burn.

4. Determine the extent of the burn. This means estimating how much body surface area the burn covers. A rough guide known as the Rule of Nines assigns a percentage value to each part of an adult's body (▶Figure 4). The entire head is 9%, one complete arm is 9%, the front torso is 18%, the complete back is 18%, and each leg is 18%. The Rule of Nines must be modified to take into account the different proportions of a small child. In small

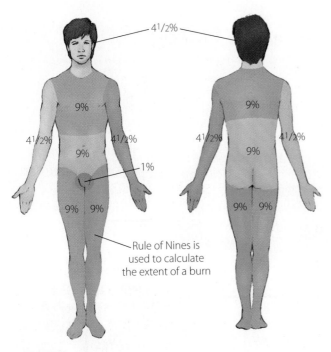

41/2%

9% 9%

41/2% 41/2% 41/2% 41/2%

9% 9%

1%

9% 9% 9% 9%

Rule of Nines is
used to calculate
the extent of a burn

Figure 4 Rule of Nines

Caution:

DO NOT remove clothing stuck to the skin—
pulling will further damage the skin.

DO NOT forget to remove jewelry as soon as
possible—swelling could make jewelry difficult
to remove later.

children and infants, the head accounts for 18% and
each leg is 14%.

For small or scattered burns, use the rule of the
palm. The victim's hand, excluding the fingers and
the thumb, represents about 1% of his or her total
body surface. Estimate the *unburned* area in number
of hands.

5. Determine what parts of the body are burned.
Burns on the face, hands, feet, and genitals are more
severe than on other body parts. A circumferential
burn (one that goes around a finger, toe, arm, leg,
neck, or chest) is considered more severe than a
noncircumferential one because it can have con-
striction and tourniquet effects on circulation and,
in some cases, breathing. All these burns require
medical care.

6. Determine if other injuries or preexisting medical
problems exist or if the victim is elderly (over 55) or

very young (under five). A medical problem or be-
longing to one of those age groups increases a
burn's severity.

7. Determine the burn's severity ▼Table 1 . This
forms the basis for how to treat the burned victim.
Most burns are minor, occur at home, and can be
managed outside a medical setting. Seek medical
attention for all moderate and severe burns, as
classified by the ABA, or if any of the following
conditions applies:

- The victim is under 5 or over 55 years of age.
- The victim has difficulty breathing.
- Other injuries exist.

Table 1: Burn Severity

Minor Burns

First-degree burn covering less than 50% BSA* in adults
(face, hands, feet, or genitals not burned)

Second-degree burn covering less than 15% BSA in adults

Second-degree burn covering less than 10% BSA in
children/elderly persons

Third-degree burn covering less than 2% BSA in adults
(face, hands, feet, or genitals not burned)

Moderate Burns

First-degree burn covering more than 50% BSA in adults

Second-degree burn covering 15% to 30% BSA in adults

Second-degree burn covering 10% to 20% BSA in
children/elderly persons

Third-degree burn covering 2% to 10% BSA in adults
(face, hands, or feet not burned)

Critical Burns

First-degree burn covering more than 70% BSA

Second-degree burn covering more than 30% BSA in adults

Second-degree burn covering more than 20% BSA in
children/elderly persons

Third-degree burn covering more than 10% BSA in adults

Third-degree burn covering more than 2% BSA in
children/elderly persons or any part of the face, hands, feet
or genitals

Also most inhalation injuries, electrical injuries, and burns
accompanied by major trauma or significant preexisting
conditions

*BSA = body surface area
Source: Adapted from the American Burn Association categorization

THERMAL BURNS

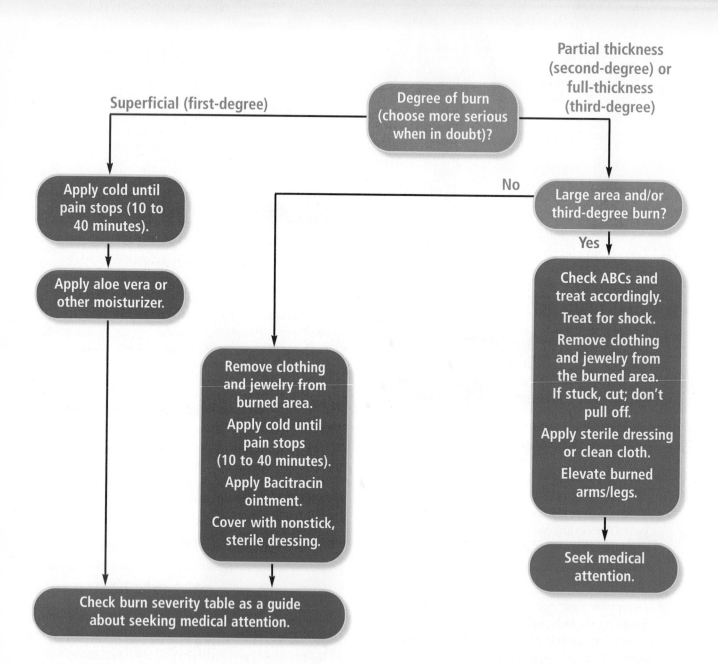

Degree of burn (choose more serious when in doubt)?

Superficial (first-degree)

Partial thickness (second-degree) or full-thickness (third-degree)

Apply cold until pain stops (10 to 40 minutes).

Apply aloe vera or other moisturizer.

No

Large area and/or third-degree burn?

Yes

Remove clothing and jewelry from burned area.

Apply cold until pain stops (10 to 40 minutes).

Apply Bacitracin ointment.

Cover with nonstick, sterile dressing.

Check ABCs and treat accordingly.

Treat for shock.

Remove clothing and jewelry from the burned area. If stuck, cut; don't pull off.

Apply sterile dressing or clean cloth.

Elevate burned arms/legs.

Seek medical attention.

Check burn severity table as a guide about seeking medical attention.

- An electrical injury exists.
- The face, hands, feet, or genitals are burned.
- Child abuse is suspected.
- The surface area of a second-degree burn is greater than 15% of the body surface area.
- The burn is third-degree.

Burn Care

Burn care aims to reduce pain, protect against infection, and prevent evaporation.

Care of First-Degree Burns

1. Immerse the burned area in cold water or apply a wet, cold cloth to reduce pain (▼Figure 5). Apply cold until the part is pain free both in and out of the water (usually in 10 minutes, but it may take up to 45 minutes). Cold also stops the burn from progressing into deeper tissue. If cold water is unavailable, use any cold drinkable liquid to reduce the temperature of the burned skin.
2. Give ibuprofen to relieve pain and inflammation. Give children acetaminophen.
3. After the burn cools, apply an aloe vera gel or an inexpensive skin moisturizer lotion to keep the skin moistened and to reduce itching and peeling. Aloe vera has antimicrobial properties and is an effective analgesic.
4. Keep a burned arm or leg elevated.

Figure 5   Immerse the burn in cold water.

Cool burn with cold water until pain is relieved.

Cooling usually takes 10–45 minutes.

Caution:

DO NOT apply cold to more than 20% of an adult's body surface (10% for children); widespread cooling can cause hypothermia. Burn victims lose large amounts of heat and water.

DO NOT apply salve, ointment, grease, butter, cream, spray, home remedy, or any other coating on a burn until after it cools. Such coatings are unsterile and can lead to infection. They also can seal in heat, causing further damage.

Care of Small Second-Degree Burns (<20% BSA)

1. Follow steps 1 and 2 of First-Degree Burn care.
2. After the burn cools, apply a thin layer of Bacitracin ointment. Topical antibiotic therapy like Bacitracin does not sterilize a wound, but it does decrease the number of bacteria to a level that can be controlled by the body's defense mechanisms and prevents the entrance of bacteria.
3. Cover the burn with a dry, nonsticking, sterile dressing or a clean cloth. Covering the burn reduces the amount of pain by keeping air from the exposed nerve endings. The main purpose of a dressing over a burn is to keep the burn clean, prevent moisture loss through evaporation, and reduce pain. If toes or fingers have been burned, place dry dressings between them.
4. Have the victim drink as much water as possible without becoming nauseous.

Caution:

DO NOT cool more than 20% of an adult's body surface area (10% for a child) except to extinguish flames.

DO NOT break any blisters. Intact blisters serve as excellent burn dressings. Cover a ruptured blister with Bacitracin ointment and a dry, sterile dressing.

CHEMICAL BURNS

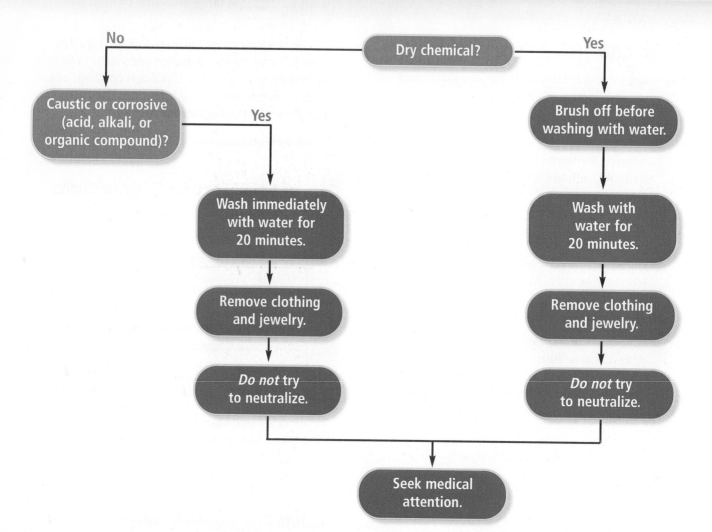

Care of Large Second-Degree Burns (>20% BSA)

Do not apply cold because it may cause hypothermia.

1. Follows steps 2 through 4 of Small Second-Degree Burn care (<20% BSA).

2. Seek medical attention.

Care of Third-Degree Burns

1. Cover the burn with a dry, nonsticking, sterile dressing or a clean cloth.

2. Treat the victim for shock by elevating the legs and keeping the victim warm with a clean sheet or blanket.

3. Seek medical attention.

Chemical Burns

A chemical burn is the result of a caustic or corrosive substance touching the skin (▼Figure 6). Because chemicals continue to "burn" as long as they are in contact with the skin, they should be removed from the victim as rapidly as possible.

First aid is the same for all chemical burns, except a few specific ones for which a chemical neutralizer has to be used. Alkalis such as drain cleaners cause more serious burns than acids such as battery acid because they penetrate deeper and remain active longer. Organic compounds such as petroleum products are also capable of burning.

Figure 6 Chemical burn from sulfuric acid

Caution:

DO NOT apply water under high pressure—it will drive the chemical deeper into the tissue.

DO NOT try to neutralize a chemical even if you know which chemical is involved—heat may be produced, resulting in more damage. Some product labels for neutralizing may be wrong. Save the container or the label for the chemical's name.

What to Do

1. Immediately remove the chemical by flushing the area with water (▼Figure 7). If available, use a hose or a shower. Brush dry powder chemicals from the skin *before* flushing, unless large amounts of water are immediately available. Water may activate a dry chemical and cause more damage to the skin. Take precautions to protect yourself from exposure to the chemical.

2. Remove the victim's contaminated clothing and jewelry while flushing with water. Clothing can hold chemicals, allowing them to continue to burn as long as they are in contact with the skin.

3. Flush for 20 minutes all chemical burns (skin, eyes). Washing with large amounts of water dilutes the chemical concentration and washes it away.

4. Cover the burned area with a dry, sterile dressing or, for large areas, a clean pillowcase.

5. Seek medical attention immediately for all chemical burns.

Figure 7 Flooding a chemical burn

ELECTRICAL BURNS

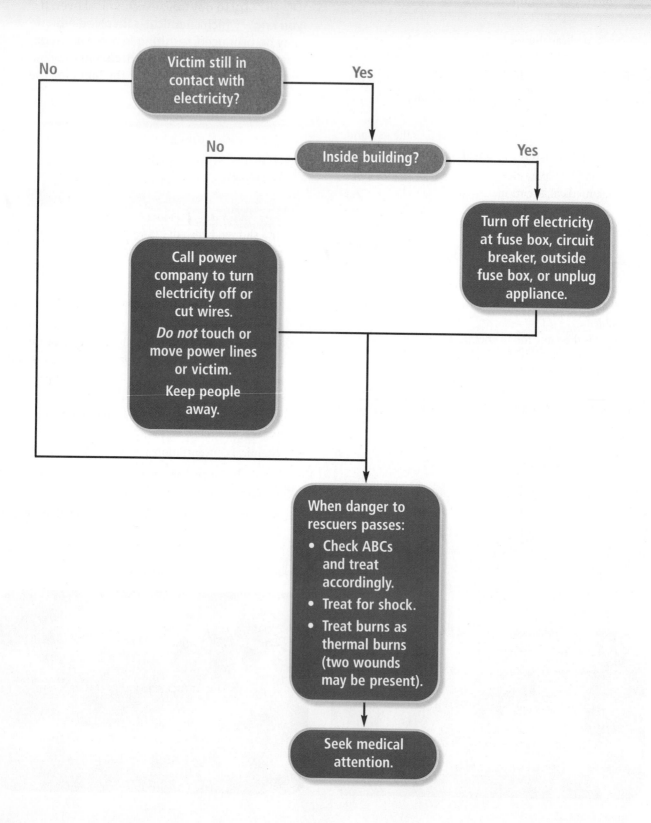

Victim still in contact with electricity?

No → Yes

Inside building?

No → Yes

Turn off electricity at fuse box, circuit breaker, outside fuse box, or unplug appliance.

Call power company to turn electricity off or cut wires.

***Do not* touch or move power lines or victim.**

Keep people away.

When danger to rescuers passes:
- Check ABCs and treat accordingly.
- Treat for shock.
- Treat burns as thermal burns (two wounds may be present).

Seek medical attention.

Electrical Burns

Even a mild electrical shock can cause serious internal injuries. A current of 1,000 volts or more is considered high voltage, but even the 110 volts found in ordinary household current can be deadly ▼Figures 8A and 8B.

There are three types of electrical injuries: thermal burn (flame), arc burn (flash), and true electrical injury (contact). A *thermal burn* (flame) results when clothing or objects in direct contact with the skin are ignited by an electrical current. These injuries are caused by the flames produced by the electrical current and not by the passage of the electrical current or arc.

An *arc burn* (flash) occurs when electricity jumps, or arcs, from one spot to another. The electrical current does not pass through the body. Although the duration of the flash may be brief, it usually causes extensive superficial injuries.

A *true electrical injury* (contact) happens when an electric current truly passes through the body. This type of injury is characterized by an entrance wound and an exit wound. The important factor in this type of injury is that the surface injury may be just the tip of the iceberg. High-voltage electrical currents passing through the body may disrupt the normal heart rhythm and cause cardiac arrest, burns, and other injuries.

During an electric shock, electricity enters the body at the point of contact and travels along the path of least resistance (nerves and blood vessels). The major damage occurs inside the body—the outside burn may appear small. Usually, the electricity exits where the body touches a surface or comes in contact with a ground (eg, a metal object). Sometimes, a victim has more than one exit site.

What to Do

1. Make sure the area is safe. Unplug, disconnect, or turn off the power. If that is impossible, call the power company or EMS for help.
2. Check ABCs.
3. If the victim fell, check for a spinal injury.
4. Treat the victim for shock.
5. Seek medical attention immediately. Electrical injuries usually require burn center care.

Contact With a Power Line (Outdoors)

If the electric shock is from contact with a downed power line, the power *must* be turned off before a rescuer approaches anyone who may be in contact with the wire.

If you can safely reach the victim, do not attempt to move any wires, even with wooden poles, tools with wood handles, or tree branches. Do not use objects with a high moisture content and certainly not metal objects. Do not attempt to move downed wires at all unless you are trained and are equipped with tools that can handle the high voltage.

Wait until trained personnel with the proper equipment can cut the wires or disconnect them. Prevent bystanders from entering the danger area.

Contact Inside Buildings

Most electrical burns that occur indoors are caused by faulty electrical equipment or careless use of electrical appliances. Turn off the electricity at the circuit breaker, fuse box, or outside switch box or unplug the appliance if the plug is undamaged. Do not touch the appliance or the victim until the current is off.

Once there is no danger to rescuers, first aid can begin.

Figure 8A Electrical burn exit wound on toe

Meeting OSHA Guidelines

This chapter covers the following OSHA Guidelines for First Aid training:

- Section IV. A. 4a. Principles and first aid intervention for assessing the severity of the burn including first degree, second degree, and third degree burns.
- Section IV. A. 4b. Differentiating between the types of third degree burns (thermal, electrical, and chemical) and their specific interventions, including chemical burns, and the use of specific chemicals in the workplace that may cause them.

Learning Activities

Thermal (Heat) Burns

Directions: Circle Yes if you agree with the statement, and circle No if you disagree.

Yes   No   **1.** Relieve pain and tissue damage from a burn by holding the part in a sink filled with running cold water.

 No   **2.** Pain and inflammation can be relieved with ibuprofen in those who can tolerate these over-the-counter medications.

 No   **3.** Later, a layer of antibiotic ointment or aloe vera gel can be applied on first- and second-degree burns.

Yes   No   **4.** Butter can be effective on first- and second-degree burns.

Scenario: Tracy is boiling water to make hot chocolate in the office kitchen. She reaches across the stove for a cup. The sleeve of her blouse touches the flame of the gas burner and ignites, sending fire racing up her arm. Her screams bring you and others racing into the kitchen. She has second-degree burns on about 7% of her body. What should you do?

_____

_____

Chemical Burns

Yes   No   **1.** When washing chemicals off the body, flush with water for at least five minutes.

Yes   No   **2.** When washing chemicals off the body, use high pressure water.

Yes   No   **3.** Do not try to neutralize a chemical because more damage may result.

Yes   No   **4.** Brush dry powder chemicals from the skin before flushing unless large amounts of water are immediately available.

Scenario: Tim is a 28-year-old man using a caustic drain cleaner to unclog a bathroom sink. Fifteen minutes after applying the chemical, he runs water into the sink, but the drain remains clogged. He then ignores the instructions on the drain cleaner package and uses a plunger to clear the drain. The solution in the sink splashes on his arm. What should you do?

_____

_____

Electrical Burns

    1. If a victim is in contact with an outdoor electrical wire, try to move it with a wooden pole or handle.

Yes   No   **2.** If the victim is inside a building, turn off the electricity at the fuse box, circuit-breaker, outside switch box, or unplug the appliance.

Scenario: Steve is trimming hedges using an old electric hedge trimmer, which is falling apart, but works. Because the three-pronged grounding plug is a little wobbly, Steve connects it to a two-pronged adapter, plugs the adapter into an outlet, and starts working on the hedges along a metal chain-link fence. Things are going well until Steve leans against the fence for support, and a powerful electric current shoots through his body, causing him to fall over. When you arrive, he is motionless. What do you do?

_____

Chapter 9

Head and Spinal Injuries

Head Injuries

Head injury is a broadly used term. Different types of head injuries include scalp wounds, skull fractures, and brain injuries. Neck and spine injuries can be present in head-injured patients.

Scalp Wounds

A bleeding scalp wound does not affect the blood supply to the brain. The brain obtains its blood supply from arteries in the neck, not the scalp. A severe scalp wound may have an accompanying skull fracture, impaled object, or spinal injury.

What to Do

1. Wear medical exam gloves.
2. Control bleeding by gently applying direct pressure with a dry sterile dressing. If the dressing becomes blood-filled, do not remove it. Add another dressing on top of the first one.
3. If you suspect a skull fracture, apply pressure around the edges of the wound and over a broad area rather than on the center of the wound. Use a doughnut (ring) pad around the area.
4. Keep the head and shoulders slightly elevated to help control bleeding if you do not suspect a spinal injury.

Caution:

DO NOT remove an embedded object; instead stabilize it in place with bulky dressings. If you suspect a skull fracture, do not clean a scalp wound or irrigate it because the fluid can carry debris and bacteria into the brain.

HEAD INJURIES

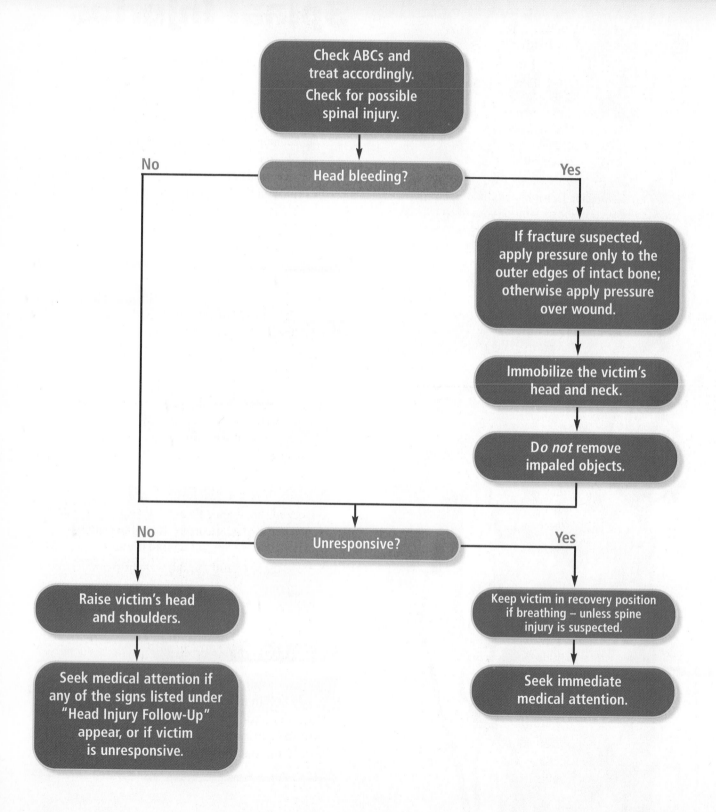

Check ABCs and treat accordingly. Check for possible spinal injury.

Head bleeding?

No

Yes

If fracture suspected, apply pressure only to the outer edges of intact bone; otherwise apply pressure over wound.

Immobilize the victim's head and neck.

Do *not* remove impaled objects.

Unresponsive?

No

Yes

Raise victim's head and shoulders.

Keep victim in recovery position if breathing – unless spine injury is suspected.

Seek medical attention if any of the signs listed under "Head Injury Follow-Up" appear, or if victim is unresponsive.

Seek immediate medical attention.

Skull Fracture

What to Look For

It is difficult to determine a skull fracture except by x-ray unless the skull deformity is severe. Signs and symptoms of a skull fracture include the following:

- Pain at the point of injury
- Deformity of the skull
- Bleeding coming from the ears or nose
- A clear, pink, watery fluid known as cerebrospinal fluid (CSF) leaking from an ear or the nose. A drop of CSF on a handkerchief, pillowcase, or other light-colored cloth will resemble a target, with a pink ring around a slightly blood-tinged center; this is called the "halo sign" or "ring sign."
- Discoloration around the eyes ("raccoon eyes") appearing several hours after the injury
- Discoloration behind an ear (known as "Battle's sign") appearing several hours after the injury
- Unequal sized pupils
- Profuse scalp bleeding if skin is broken. A scalp wound may expose the skull or brain tissue
- Penetrating wound (eg, from a bullet) or impaled object

What to Do

1. Monitor ABCs.
2. Cover wounds with a sterile dressing.
3. Stabilize the victim's neck against movement.
4. To control bleeding, apply pressure around the edges of the wound, not directly on it.

Brain Injuries

When the head is struck with sufficient force, the brain bounces against the inside of the skull.

The brain, like other body tissue, will swell from bleeding. Unlike other tissues, however, the brain is confined in the skull where there is little space for swelling. Therefore, swelling of brain tissue or accumulation of blood inside the skull compresses the brain and increases the pressure inside the skull, which interferes with brain functioning.

What to Look For

The following are frequently observed signs and symptoms of a concussion, according to the American Academy of Neurology and the Brain Injury Association:*

1. Confused facial expression
2. Slow to answer questions or follow instruction
3. Easily distracted and unable to follow through with normal activities
4. Walking in the wrong direction; unaware of time, date, and place
5. Making disjointed or incomprehensible statements
6. Stumbling, inability to walk straight line

---

*Source: Adapted from Management of Concussion in Sports, American Academy of Neurology and Brain Injury Association

7. Distraught, crying for no apparent reason

8. Asking the same question even though it has was already been answered, or unable to memorize and recall three words or three objects in sequence in five minutes

9. Coma, unresponsiveness

What to Do

1. Seek immediate medical attention for all brain-injury victims.

2. Suspect a spinal injury in an unresponsive victim until proved otherwise.

3. Monitor ABCs.

4. Control bleeding by covering wounds with sterile dressings as a barrier against infection. If you suspect a skull fracture, apply pressure around the wound edges, not directly on the wound.

5. Brain-injury victims tend to vomit. Rolling the victim onto his or her side while stabilizing the neck against movement will help drain vomit and keep the airway open.

Unfortunately, there is little a first aider can do for a brain injury. The victim must be transported to the care of a neurosurgeon.

Caution:

DO NOT stop the flow of blood or CSF from the ears or nose. Blocking either flow could increase pressure inside the skull.

DO NOT elevate the legs—that might increase pressure on the brain.

DO NOT clean an open skull injury—infection of the brain may result.

Eye Injuries

Eye injuries can involve minor conditions such as a foreign object such as dirt in the eye. But they can also involve more severe injuries that can compromise sight if not cared for immediately. Do not assume that any eye injury is innocent. When in doubt, seek medical attention immediately.

Penetrating Eye Injuries

Penetrating eye injuries are severe injuries that result when a sharp object such as a knife or a needle penetrates

the eye and then is withdrawn or when pieces from a tool enter the eye and lodge there as foreign bodies.

What to Do

1. Seek immediate medical attention. Any penetrating eye injury should be managed in the hospital.

2. Stabilize any object. Stabilize a long protruding object with bulky dressings or clean cloths. You can place a protective paper cup or a piece of cardboard folded (▶Figure 1) into a cone over the affected eye to prevent bumping of the object. For short objects, surround the eye without touching the object with a doughnut-shaped (ring) pad held on with a roller bandage.

3. Cover the undamaged eye. Most experts suggest that the undamaged eye should be covered to prevent sympathetic eye movement (ie, the injured eye moves when the undamaged one does) and aggravating the injury. Remember that the victim is unable to see when both eyes are covered and may be anxious. Make sure you explain everything you are doing.

Caution:

DO NOT wash out the eye with water.

DO NOT try to remove an object stuck in the eye.

DO NOT press on an injured eyeball or penetrating object.

Blows to the Eye

Blows to the eye can be minor to sight-threatening (▶Figure 2).

What to Do

1. Apply an ice pack immediately for about 15 minutes to reduce pain and swelling. Do not exert any pressure on the eye.

2. Seek medical attention immediately if there is pain, reduced vision, or discoloration (a black eye).

Cuts of the Eye or Lid (▶Figure 3)
What to Do

1. Bandage both eyes lightly.

2. Seek medical attention immediately.

Figures 1A, 1B, and 1C Protecting a long penetrating object against movement (using paper cup).

Chemical Burns of the Eye

Chemical burns of the eyes are extremely sight-threatening. First aid may determine the fate of the eye and vision.

Alkalis cause greater damage than acids because they penetrate deeper and continue to burn longer. Common alkalis include drain cleaners, cleaning agents, ammonia, cement, plaster, and caustic soda. Common acids include hydrochloric acid, nitric acid, sulfuric (battery) acid, and acetic acid.

Because damage can happen in 1 to 5 minutes, the chemical must be removed immediately.

Figure 2 Blow to the eye

Figure 3 Lacerated eyelid

What to Do

1. Use your fingers to keep the eye open as wide as possible.
2. Flush the eye with water immediately (▼**Figure 4**). If possible, use warm water. If water is not available, use any nonirritating liquid.
   - Hold the victim's head under a faucet or pour water into the eye from any clean container for 20 minutes, continuously and gently. It is impossible to use too much water on these injuries.

Figure 4 Flushing eye for chemical burn

EYE INJURIES

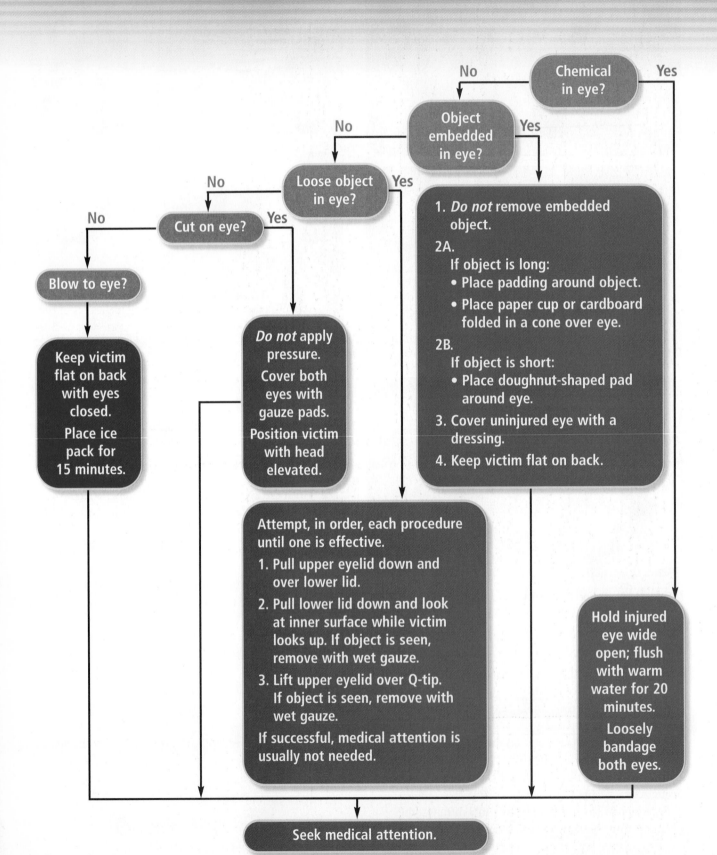

Chemical in eye?
No → / Yes →

Object embedded in eye?
No → / Yes →

Loose object in eye?
No → / Yes →

Cut on eye?
No → / Yes →

Blow to eye?

Keep victim flat on back with eyes closed.
Place ice pack for 15 minutes.

Do not apply pressure.
Cover both eyes with gauze pads.
Position victim with head elevated.

1. *Do not* remove embedded object.
2A.
   If object is long:
   • Place padding around object.
   • Place paper cup or cardboard folded in a cone over eye.
2B.
   If object is short:
   • Place doughnut-shaped pad around eye.
3. Cover uninjured eye with a dressing.
4. Keep victim flat on back.

Attempt, in order, each procedure until one is effective.
1. Pull upper eyelid down and over lower lid.
2. Pull lower lid down and look at inner surface while victim looks up. If object is seen, remove with wet gauze.
3. Lift upper eyelid over Q-tip. If object is seen, remove with wet gauze.
If successful, medical attention is usually not needed.

Hold injured eye wide open; flush with warm water for 20 minutes.
Loosely bandage both eyes.

Seek medical attention.

- Irrigate from the nose side of the eye toward the outside, to avoid flushing material into the other eye.
- Tell the victim to roll the eyeball as much as possible to help wash out the eye.

3. Loosely bandage both eyes with cold, wet dressings.

4. Seek immediate medical attention.

Caution:

DO NOT try to neutralize the chemical. Water usually is readily available and better for eye irrigation.

DO NOT bandage eye tightly.

Eye Knocked Out

A blow to the eye can knock it from its socket.

What to Do

1. Cover the eye loosely with a sterile dressing that has been moistened with clean water. Do not try to push the eyeball back into the socket.

2. Protect the injured eye with a paper cup, a piece of cardboard folded into a cone, or a doughnut-shaped pad made from a roller gauze bandage or a cravat bandage.

3. Cover the undamaged eye.

4. Seek medical attention immediately.

Foreign Objects in Eye

Try one or more of the following techniques, beginning with the first step (▶**Figure 5**).

What to Do

1. Lift the upper lid over the lower lid, allowing the lashes to brush the object off the inside of the upper lid. Have the victim blink a few times and let the eye move the object out. If the object remains, keep the eye closed.

2. Try flushing the object out by rinsing the eye gently with warm water. Hold the eyelid open and tell the victim to move the eye as it is rinsed.

3. Examine the lower lid by pulling it down gently. If you can see the object, remove it with a moistened sterile gauze or clean cloth.

Figure 5   Removing foreign object from the eye

a. If tears or gentle flushing do not remove object, gently pull lower lid down. Remove an object by gently flushing with lukewarm water or a wet sterile gauze.

b. Fold the lid over the swab or matchstick. Remove an object by gently flushing with lukewarm water or a wet sterile gauze.

4. Examine the upper lid by grasping the lashes of the upper lid, placing a match stick or cotton-tipped swab across the upper lid and rolling the lid upward over the stick or swab. If you can see the object, remove it with a moistened sterile gauze or clean cloth or flush it out.

Caution:

DO NOT allow the victim to rub the eye.

DO NOT try to remove an embedded foreign object.

DO NOT use dry cotton (cotton balls or cotton-tipped swabs) or instruments (eg, tweezers) on an eye.

Eye Burns from Light

Burns can result if a person looks at a source of ultraviolet light (eg, sunlight, arc welding, bright snow, tanning lamps). Severe pain begins 1 to 6 hours after exposure.

What to Do

1. Cover both eyes with cold, wet packs. Tell the victim not to rub the eyes.

2. Have the victim rest in a darkened room. Do not allow light to reach the victim's eyes.

3. Give pain medication if needed.

4. Call an ophthalmologist for medical advice.

DENTAL INJURIES

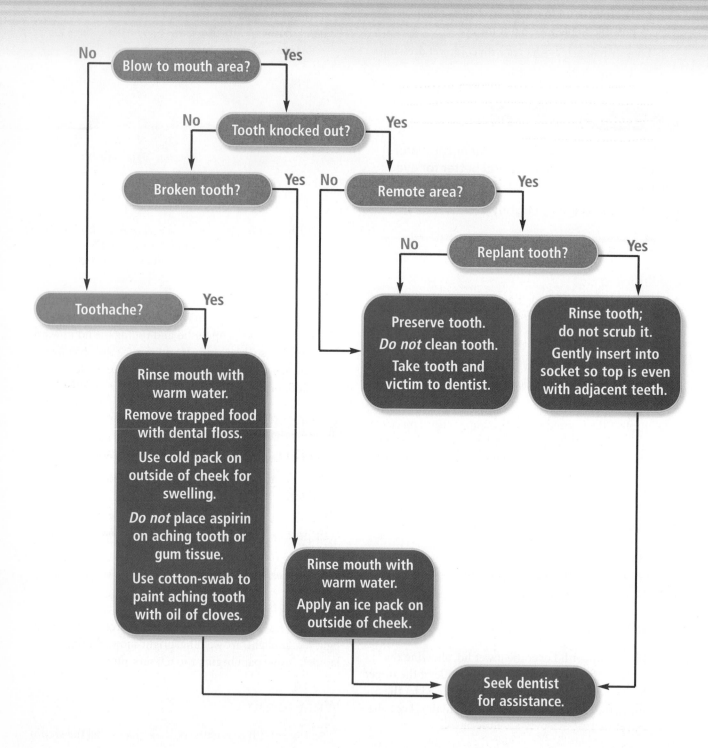

No — Blow to mouth area? — Yes

No — Tooth knocked out? — Yes

Broken tooth? — Yes

No — Remote area? — Yes

No — Replant tooth? — Yes

Toothache? — Yes

Rinse mouth with warm water.
Remove trapped food with dental floss.
Use cold pack on outside of cheek for swelling.
Do not **place aspirin on aching tooth or gum tissue.**
Use cotton-swab to paint aching tooth with oil of cloves.

Preserve tooth.
Do not **clean tooth.**
Take tooth and victim to dentist.

Rinse tooth; do not scrub it.
Gently insert into socket so top is even with adjacent teeth.

Rinse mouth with warm water.
Apply an ice pack on outside of cheek.

Seek dentist for assistance.

Nose Injuries

Nosebleeds

There are two types of nosebleeds:

- *Anterior (front of nose)* is the most common type (90%). Blood comes out of the nose through one nostril.

- *Posterior (back of nose)* type involves massive bleeding backward into the mouth or down the back of the throat. A posterior nosebleed is serious and requires medical attention.

Caution:

DO NOT allow the victim to tilt the head backward.

DO NOT probe the nose with a cotton-tipped swab.

DO NOT move the victim's head and neck if a spinal injury is suspected.

What to Do

1. Place the victim in a seated position.

2. Keep the victim's head tilted slightly forward so blood can run out the front of the nose, not down the back of the throat, which can cause choking, nausea, or vomiting.

3. Pinch (or have the victim pinch) all the soft parts of the nose together between the thumb and two fingers with steady pressure for five minutes. While pinching the nostrils, push the pinched parts against the bones of the face.

4. If bleeding persists, have the victim gently blow the nose to remove any irregular clots and excess blood and to minimize sneezing. This allows new clots to form. If available, spray the nose four times on each side with a decongestant spray (Afrin™, Neo-Synephrin™), then pinch the nostrils again for five minutes.

5. Apply an ice pack over the nose and cheeks to help control bleeding—especially if caused by a blow to the nose.

6. Seek medical attention if any of the following applies:

   - The nostril pinching and other methods do not stop the bleeding.

   - You suspect a posterior nosebleed.

   - The victim has high blood pressure or is taking anticoagulants (blood thinners) or large doses of aspirin.

   - Bleeding happens after a blow to the nose, and you suspect a broken nose.

Broken Nose

1. Seek medical attention.

2. Treat a nosebleed as described above.

3. Apply an ice pack to the nose for 15 minutes. Do not try to straighten a crooked nose.

Dental Injuries

Because dental emergencies generally cause considerable pain and anxiety, managing them promptly can provide great relief to the victim.

Knocked-Out Tooth

A knocked-out tooth is a common dental emergency (▼Figure 6). More than 90% of the two million teeth knocked out each year in the United States could be saved with proper treatment.

Emergency care for knocked-out teeth has changed dramatically in recent years. The first question you want to ask in this situation is, "Where is the tooth?" Time is crucial for successful reimplantation. After a tooth is knocked out, ligament fiber fragments remain attached to the tooth and to the bone in the socket. However, the ligament fibers begin to die soon after the injury. Therefore, it is important to prevent the tooth from drying. Moisture alone is not sufficient to preserve the tooth's ligament fibers. Steps must be taken both to prevent the tooth from becoming dehydrated and to protect the ligament fibers from damage.

Figure 6 Tooth knocked out

1. Have the victim rinse his or her month, and put a rolled gauze pad in the socket to control bleeding.

2. Find the tooth and handle it by the crown, not the root, to minimize damage to the ligament fibers.

3. The best place for a knocked-out tooth is its socket. A tooth can often be successfully reimplanted if it is replaced in its socket within 30 minutes after the injury; the odds of successful reimplantation decrease about 1% for every minute the tooth is absent from the socket. If you feel you can do this without causing more injury to the victim, gently rinse any debris from the tooth and try to place the tooth into the socket, using adjacent teeth as a guide. Apply pressure on the tooth so the top is even with the adjacent teeth.

Immediate reinsertion is not always possible, however. The victim may be reluctant to put the knocked-out tooth back into its socket, especially if it has fallen on the ground and is covered with debris. Or the tooth may repeatedly fall out, putting the victim at risk of inhaling or swallowing it. In victims with multiple trauma, the presence of more serious injuries may prevent reinsertion.

When immediate reinsertion is not possible, the tooth should be transported in a moist environment. The best transport medium is the Save-a-Tooth Kit™. Its use extends the viability of the ligament fibers for 6 to 12 hours. If this is not available, cool milk can be used.

Some experts recommend that the tooth be placed in the victim's mouth to keep it moist until dental treatment is available. This method, although convenient, presents the risk of the tooth's being accidentally swallowed, especially by children.

4. Take the victim and the tooth to a dentist immediately even if it has been reinserted.

Dental Emergency Procedures

Bitten Lip or Tongue	Clean the area gently with a cloth and apply cold compresses to reduce any swelling. If the bleeding does not stop, go to a hospital emergency room immediately.
Broken Tooth	Rinse your mouth with warm water to clean the area. Use cold compresses on the area to keep any swelling down. Call your dentist immediately.
Jaw–Possibly Broken	Apply cold compresses to control swelling. Go to your dentist or a hospital emergency department immediately.
Knocked-Out Tooth	Hold the tooth by the crown and rinse off the root of the tooth in water if it is dirty. Do not scrub it or remove any attached tissue fragments. If possible, gently insert the tooth in its socket. If that is not possible, put the tooth in a cup of milk and get to the dentist as quickly as possible. Remember to take the tooth with you!
Objects Caught Between Teeth	Try to gently remove the object with dental floss; avoid cutting the gums. Never use a sharp instrument to remove any object that is stuck between your teeth. If you cannot dislodge the object using dental floss, contact your dentist.
Toothache	Rinse your mouth with warm water to clean it out. Gently use dental floss or an interdental cleaner to ensure that there is not food or other debris caught between the teeth. Never put aspirin of any other painkiller against the gums near the aching tooth because it may burn the gum tissue. If the pain persists, contact your dentist.

Source: Copyright by the American Dental Association; reprinted with permission.

Broken Tooth ▼Figure 7
What to Do

1. Gently clean dirt and blood from the injured area with a sterile gauze pad or a clean cloth and warm water.
2. Apply an ice pack to the face in the area of the injured tooth to decrease swelling.
3. If you suspect a jaw fracture, stabilize the jaw by wrapping a bandage under the chin and over the top of the head.
4. Seek a dentist immediately.

Figure 7 Broken teeth

Toothache

The tooth will be sensitive to heat and cold. Identify the diseased tooth by tapping the area with a spoon handle or similar object. A diseased tooth will hurt.

What to Do

1. Rinse the mouth with warm water to clean it out.
2. Use dental floss to remove any food that might be trapped between the teeth.
3. Give the victim pain medication such as ibuprofen.
4. Seek a dentist immediately.

Spinal Injuries

Head injuries serve as a clue to possible spinal injuries because the head may have been moved suddenly in one or more directions, damaging the spine.

What to Look For ▶Skill Scan

- Painful movement of the arms or legs
- Numbness, tingling, weakness, or burning sensation in the arms or legs
- Loss of bowel or bladder control
- Paralysis of the arms or legs
- Deformity (odd-looking angle of the victim's head and neck)

- Check a responsive victim by using techniques shown in the Skill Scan: *Checking for Spinal Injuries* on page 75.

If the victim is unresponsive, do the following:

- Look for cuts, bruises, and deformities.
- Test responses by pinching the victim's hand (either palm or back of the hand) and bare foot (sole or top of the foot). No reaction could mean spinal damage.
- Ask bystanders what happened. If you still are not sure about a possible spinal injury, assume the victim has one until it is proved otherwise.

What to Do

1. Stabilize the victim against any movement ▼Figure 8 .
2. Check ABC.

Figure 8 Stabilize head against movement.

Meeting OSHA Guidelines

This chapter covers the following OSHA Guidelines for First Aid training:

- Section IV. B. 1a. Principles and first aid intervention of injuries to the head and neck, including skull fractures, concussions, and mental status assessments, with particular attention to temporary loss of consciousness and the need for referral to a physician.
- Section IV. B. 1b. Appropriate approach to the management of the individual who has suffered a potential neck or back injury or fracture.
- Section IV. B. 2a-c. Principles and first aid intervention of injuries to the eye, including foreign bodies, corneal abrasions, lacerations, chemical burns and the importance of flushing out the eye, and the importance of proper application of antibiotics.
- Section IV. B. 3a. Principles and first aid intervention of injuries to the nose, including nose bleeds.
- Section IV. B. 4a. Principles and first aid intervention of oral injuries, lip and tongue injuries, and broken and removed teeth. The importance of preventing inhalation of blood and teeth.

SPINAL INJURIES

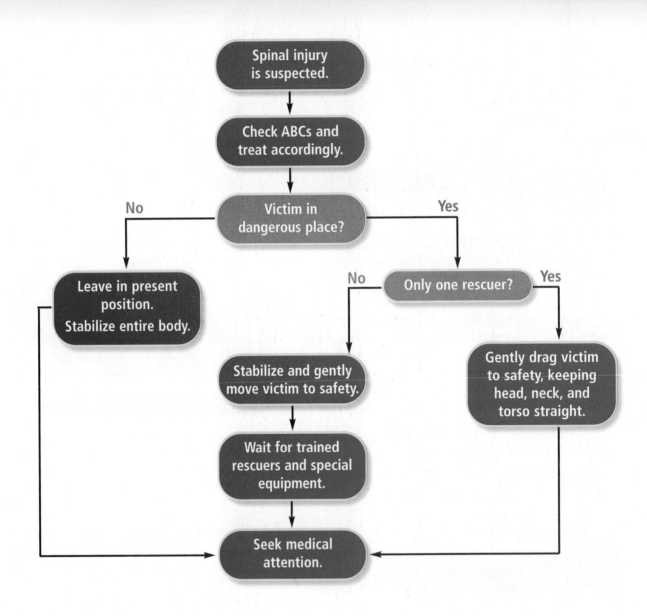

Skill Scan | Checking for Spinal Injuries

Responsive Victim—Upper Extremity Checks

1. Victim wiggles fingers.

2. Victim feels rescuer squeeze fingers.

3. Victim squeezes rescuer's hand.

Responsive Victim—Lower-Extremity Checks

1. Victim wiggles toes.

2. Victim feels rescuer squeezes toes.

3. Victim pushes foot against rescuer's hand.

Learning Activities

Head Injuries

Directions: Circle Yes if you agree with the statement, and circle No if you disagree.

Yes   No   **1.** Press around the edges of a suspected skull fracture and not directly on the wound.

Yes   No   **2.** Do NOT remove impaled (embedded) objects.

Yes   No   **3.** Head injured victims should be checked for a possible spinal injury.

Scenario: At work, you are called to help a carpenter who fell from a ladder. A bystander says that, though responsive now, the victim was previously motionless for a couple of minutes. The victim complains about a severe headache and dizziness. There is swelling on the back of his head. What should you do?

_____

Eye Injuries

Yes   No   **1.** After a blow to an eye, apply a cold pack for about 15 minutes.

Yes   No   **2.** Tears are sufficient to flush a chemical from the eye.

Yes   No   **3.** Use a clean, damp cloth to remove an object from the eyelid's surface.

Scenario: As Sam is attempting to jump-start the company car, a spark from the jump-cables ignites hydrogen gas accumulated in the battery. This causes the battery to explode. The battery cap flies off, and battery acid splashes into Sam's eyes. What should you do?

_____

Dental Injuries

Yes   No   **1.** Preserve a knocked-out tooth in mouthwash or rubbing alcohol.

Yes   No   **2.** Scrub a knocked-out tooth before taking the victim to a dentist.

Yes   No   **3.** A knocked-out tooth can be placed in milk.

Scenario: Mike, age 20, was struck in the mouth by a pipe loosely suspended from a cable. He has spit out two of his front teeth, which are lying on the ground. What should you do?

_____

Spinal Injuries

Yes   No   **1.** Do NOT move a victim with a suspected spinal injury.

Yes   No   **2.** Inability to move fingers and/or feet may indicate a spinal injury.

Yes   No   **3.** A head injury may be a reason to suspect a spinal injury.

Scenario: You heard a loud crash when a car hit a concrete median. You have done a scene survey. The driver complains of numbness and loss of feeling in both legs. What should you do?

_____

Chest, Abdominal, and Pelvic Injuries

Chest Injuries

All chest injury victims should be checked and rechecked for ABCs. A responsive chest injury victim should usually sit up or be placed with the injured side down. This position protects the uninjured side from blood inside the chest cavity and allows the uninjured side to expand.

Broken Ribs

Broken ribs usually occur along the side of the chest. The main symptom of a broken rib is pain when the victim breathes, coughs, or moves and pain at the injured site. Pain produced when squeezing the chest during the physical exam is another indication of a broken rib.

What to Do

1. Help the victim find a comfortable position. Stabilize the ribs by having the victim hold a pillow or other similar soft object against the injured area (▶Figure 1A and 1B). Or use bandages to hold the pillow in place or tie an arm over the injured area. Do not apply tight bandages around the chest because they restrict breathing. Some victims find comfort by lying on the injured side.
2. Seek medical attention.

Impaled Object in Chest
What to Do

1. Stabilize the object in place with bulky dressings (▶Figure 2A and 2B). *Do not try to remove an impaled object*—bleeding and air in the chest cavity can result.
2. Seek medical attention.

Figure 1, A–B Stabilize chest with soft object such as pillow, coat, or blanket (hold or tie).

Figure 2, A–B **A.** Stabilize penetrating object with bulky padding. **B.** Secure padding and object.

Sucking Chest Wound

A sucking chest wound results when a chest wound allows air to pass into and out of the chest cavity with each breath.

What to Do

1. Have the victim take a breath and let it out; then seal the wound with anything available to stop air from entering the chest cavity. Plastic wrap or a plastic bag works well. Tape it in place but leave one corner untaped. This creates a flutter valve to prevent air from being trapped in the chest cavity. If plastic wrap is not available, you can use your gloved hand.

2. If the victim has trouble breathing or seems to be getting worse, remove the plastic cover (or your hand) to let air escape, then reapply.

3. Seek medical attention.

CHEST INJURIES

Check ABCs and treat accordingly.

↓

Penetrating wound?

No → / Yes →

Impaled object?

No / Yes

Sucking chest wound?

No / Yes

Do not remove object. Stabilize object.

Rib fracture?

Yes

Seal wound to prevent air from entering.

Stabilize ribs and chest.

Seek medical attention.

Abdominal Injuries

Blow to the Abdomen

Examine the abdomen by gently pressing different areas of the abdomen with your fingertips. Observe for pain, tenderness, muscle tightness, or rigidity. A normal abdomen is soft and not tender when pressed.

What to Do

1. Place the victim in a comfortable position and expect vomiting. Do not give the victim any food or drink. If you are hours from a medical facility, allow the victim to suck on a clean cloth soaked in water to relieve a dry mouth.
2. Seek medical attention.

Penetrating Wound

Expect internal organs to be damaged.

What to Do

1. If the penetrating object is still in place, stabilize the object and control bleeding by using bulky dressings around it. *Do not try to remove the object.*
2. Seek medical attention.

Protruding Organs

What to Do

Position the victim with head and shoulders slightly raised, and knees bent and raised.

1. Cover protruding organs with a moistened sterile dressing or clean cloth (▶Figure 3).
2. Place a towel lightly over the dressing to help maintain warmth
3. Seek medical attention.

Figure 3 Do not reinsert protruding organs. Cover them with a moist, sterile dressing.

Pelvic Injuries

If you suspect a broken pelvis, gently press the sides of the pelvis downward and squeeze them inward at the iliac crests (upper points of the hips). A broken pelvis will be painful. Just like other injuries, if the victim is already complaining about pain, do not apply pressure.

What to Do

1. Treat the victim for shock.
2. Place padding between the victim's thighs, then tie the victim's knees and ankles together. If the knees are bent, place padding under them for support.
3. Keep the victim on a firm surface.
4. Seek medical attention.

Caution:

DO NOT try to reinsert protruding organs into the abdomen—you could introduce infection or damage the intestines.

DO NOT cover the organs tightly.

DO NOT cover the organs with any material that clings or disintegrates when wet.

DO NOT give anything to eat or drink.

Meeting OSHA Guidelines

This chapter covers the following OSHA Guidelines for First Aid training:

- Section IV. B. 5a. Principles and first aid intervention of injuries to the chest, including rib fractures, flail chest, and penetrating wounds.
- Section IV. B. 6a. Principles and first aid intervention of injuries to the abdomen, including blunt injuries, penetrating injuries, and protruding organs.

ABDOMINAL INJURIES

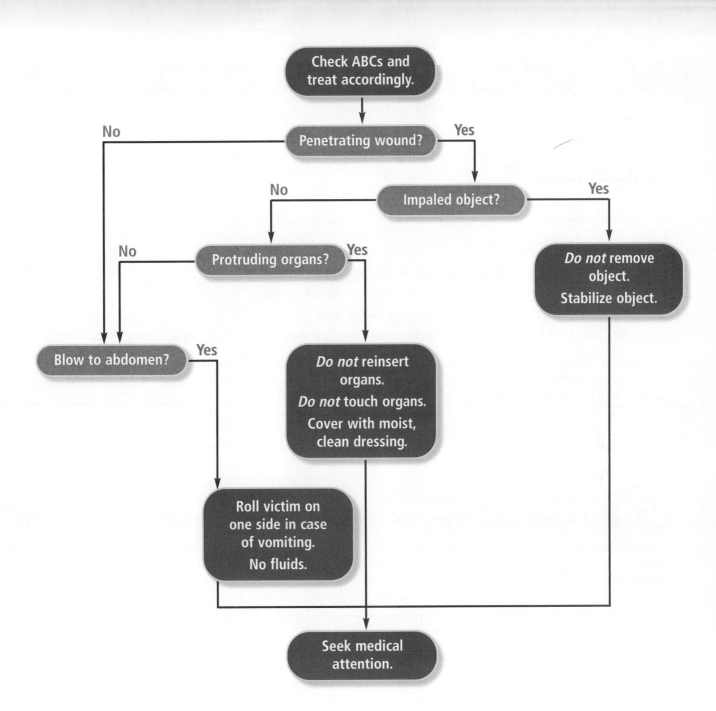

Check ABCs and treat accordingly.

Penetrating wound?

No — Yes

Impaled object?

No — Yes

Do not remove object.
Stabilize object.

Protruding organs?

No — Yes

Blow to abdomen?

Yes

Do not reinsert organs.
Do not touch organs.
Cover with moist, clean dressing.

Roll victim on one side in case of vomiting.
No fluids.

Seek medical attention.

Learning Activities

Chest Injuries

Directions: Circle Yes if you agree with the statement, and circle No if you disagree.

Yes ~~No~~   1. Stabilize a broken rib by strapping (taping) a victim's chest as tightly as possible.

~~Yes~~ No   2. Stabilize an impaled (embedded) object in the chest with bulky padding to prevent it from moving.

~~Yes~~ No   3. Cover a sucking chest wound with plastic wrap.

Scenario: An iron rod broke and stuck into a construction worker's chest as he tied the rods for a concrete foundation. You are called over to help with the injured worker and you find that the iron rod has been removed. Air is passing into and out of the victim's chest with each breath he takes. What should you do?

_____

_____

_____

Abdominal Injuries

Yes ~~No~~   1. Gently push protruding organs back through the abdominal wound.

Yes ~~No~~   2. The dressing covering exposed intestines should be kept dry.

Yes ~~No~~   3. Remove any penetrating object from the abdomen.

~~Yes~~ No   4. For a blow to the abdomen with suspected internal injuries, place the victim on his or her side.

Scenario: A 45-year-old repairman fell while carrying a replacement glass for a broken window. The new glass broke in several jagged pieces. You find him lying on his back with a blood-soaked shirt. You see a lacerated abdomen with several loops of bowel protruding through the laceration. What should you do?

_____

_____

_____

Pelvic Injuries

~~Yes~~ No   1. Keep the victim on a firm surface.

~~Yes~~ No   2. Keep the victim's knees bent and place padding between the legs.

Scenario: An older secretary slipped while on stairs and fell down five steps. She is at the bottom of the stairs lying on her side. You suspect a pelvic fracture because she is complaining about severe pain in the pelvic area. What should you do?

_____

_____

_____

Chapter 11

Bone, Joint, and Muscle Injuries

Fractures

The terms "fracture" and "broken bone" have the same meaning: a break or crack in a bone. There are two categories of fractures (▶Figure 1):

- Closed (simple) fracture (▶Figure 2). The skin is intact and no wound exists anywhere near the fracture site.

- Open (compound) fracture. The skin over the fracture has been damaged or broken (▶Figure 3). The wound may result from bone protruding through the skin or by a direct blow that cuts the skin at the time of the fracture. The bone may not always be visible in the wound.

The real problems is not the broken bones themselves but the potential injury to the vital organs next to them.

What to Look For

It may be difficult to tell if a bone is fractured. When in doubt, treat the injury as a fracture. Use the mnemonic **D-O-T-S** (deformity, open wound, tenderness, swelling) found on page 15:

- *Deformity* might not be obvious. Compare the injured part with the uninjured part on the other side.

- *Open wound* may indicate an underlying fracture.

- *Tenderness* and pain are commonly found only at the injury site. Usually, the victim will be able to point to the site of the pain. A useful procedure for detecting a fracture is to gently feel along the bone; a victim's complaint about pain or tenderness serve as a reliable sign of a fracture.

- *Swelling* caused by bleeding happens rapidly after a fracture.

Additional signs and symptoms include:

- *Loss of use* may or may not occur. The victim may refuse to use the injured part if motion produces

Closed fracture   Open fracture

Figure 1 Fractures

Figure 2A Forearm fracture

Figure 2B X-rays of victim with forearm fracture before and after setting.

Figure 3 Open tibia, fibula fracture of the leg.

pain. This is called "guarding." Sometimes, however, the victim is able to move a fractured limb with little or no pain.

- *A grating sensation* can be felt and sometimes even heard when the ends of the broken bone rub together. Do not move the injured limb in an attempt to detect it.

- *The history of the injury* can lead you to suspect a fracture whenever a serious accident has happened. The victim may have heard or felt the bone snap.

What to Do

1. Determine what happened and the location of the injury.

2. Gently remove clothing covering the injured area. Cut clothing at the seams if necessary.

3. Examine the area by looking and feeling for D-O-T-S).

   - Look at the injury site. Swelling and black-and-blue marks, which indicate that blood is escaping into the tissues, may come from either the bone end or associated muscular and blood vessel damage. Shortening or severe deformity (angulation) between the joints, deformity around the joints, shortening of the extremity, and rotation of the extremity when compared with the opposite extremity indicate a bone injury. Lacerations or even small puncture wounds near the site of a bone fracture are considered open fractures.

   - Feel the injured area. If a fracture is not obvious, gently press, touch, or feel along the length of the bone for deformities, tenderness, and swelling.

BONE INJURIES

Remove or cut away clothing over injury site.

↓

Look and feel for D-O-T-S.

↓

No ← Bleeding from open fracture? → Yes

↓

Control bleeding.
Do not push bone.
Cover wound and bone with a dressing.

↓

Check circulation, sensation, and movement (CSM).

↓

Most broken bones are minor and do not need straightening.
Apply splint.
Recheck CSM periodically.

↓

Seek medical attention.

5. Check blood flow and nerves. Use the mnemonic CSM (circulation, sensation, movement) as a way of remembering what to do (▶ **Skill Scan**).

  • *Circulation.* Feel for the radial pulse (located on the thumb side of the wrist) for an arm injury and the posterior tibial pulse (located between the inside ankle bone and the Achilles tendon) for a leg injury. A pulseless arm or leg is a significant emergency that requires immediate surgical care.

  • *Sensation.* This is the most useful sign. Lightly touch or squeeze the victim's toes or fingers and ask the victim what he or she feels. Loss of sensation is an early sign of nerve damage or spinal damage.

  • *Movement.* Inability to move develops later. Check for nerve damage by asking the victim to wiggle his or her toes or fingers. If the toes or fingers are injured, do not have the victim attempt to move them.

The major blood vessels of an extremity tend to run close to the bone. Any time a bone is broken, the adjacent blood vessels are at risk of being torn by bone fragments or pinched off between the ends of the broken bone. The tissues of the arms and legs cannot survive without a continuing blood supply for more than two or three hours. In that case seek immediate medical attention.

6. Use the RICE (rest-ice-compression-elevation) procedures (see page 89).

7. Use a splint to stabilize the fracture (see Chapter 12).

8. Seek medical attention.

Joint Injuries
Dislocations

A dislocation occurs when a joint comes apart and stays apart with the bone ends no longer in contact. The shoulders, elbows, fingers, hips, kneecaps, and ankles are the joints most frequently affected. Dislocations cause signs and symptoms similar to those of a fracture: deformity, severe pain, swelling, and the inability of the victim to move the injured joint. The main sign of a dislocation is deformity. A dislocated joint will definitely look different from an uninjured joint.

What to Do

1. Check the CSM (circulation, sensation, movement). If the end of the dislocated bone is pressing on

nerves or blood vessels, numbness or paralysis may exist below the dislocation. Always check the pulses. If there is no pulse in the injured extremity, transport the victim to a medical facility immediately.

2. Use the RICE (rest, ice, compression, elevation) procedures.

3. Use a splint to stabilize the joint in the position in which it was found (see Chapter 12).

4. Do not try to reduce the joint (put the displaced parts back into their normal positions), because nerve and blood vessel damage could result.

5. Seek medical attention to reduce the dislocation.

Sprains

A sprain is an injury to a joint in which the ligaments and other tissues are damaged by violent stretching or twisting. Attempts to move or use the joint increase the pain. The skin around the joint may be discolored because of bleeding from torn tissues. It often is difficult to distinguish between a severe sprain and a fracture, because their signs and symptoms are similar.

Treatment consists of rest, ice, compression, and elevation (RICE). It is vitally important to keep a joint from swelling by applying cold promptly; it is even more important to make the swelling recede as quickly as possible with a compression (elastic) bandage.

Muscle Injuries
Strains

A muscle strain, also known as a "pulled muscle," occurs when a muscle is stretched beyond its normal range of motion, and tears.

What to Look For

Any of the following signs and symptoms may indicate a muscle strain:

  • sharp pain
  • extreme tenderness when the area is touched
  • cavity, indentation, or bump that can be felt or seen
  • severe weakness and loss of function of the injured part
  • stiffness and pain when the victim moves the muscle

What to Do

Use the RICE procedures.

Skill Scan　Checking an Extremity's CSM

Check an Upper Extremity For:

1. Circulation—radial pulse.

2. Sensation—squeeze fingers.

3. Movement—wiggle fingers.

Check a Lower Extremity For:

1. Circulation—posterial tibial pulse.

2. Sensation—squeeze toe.

3. Movement—wiggle toes.

SPRAINS, STRAINS, CONTUSIONS, DISLOCATIONS

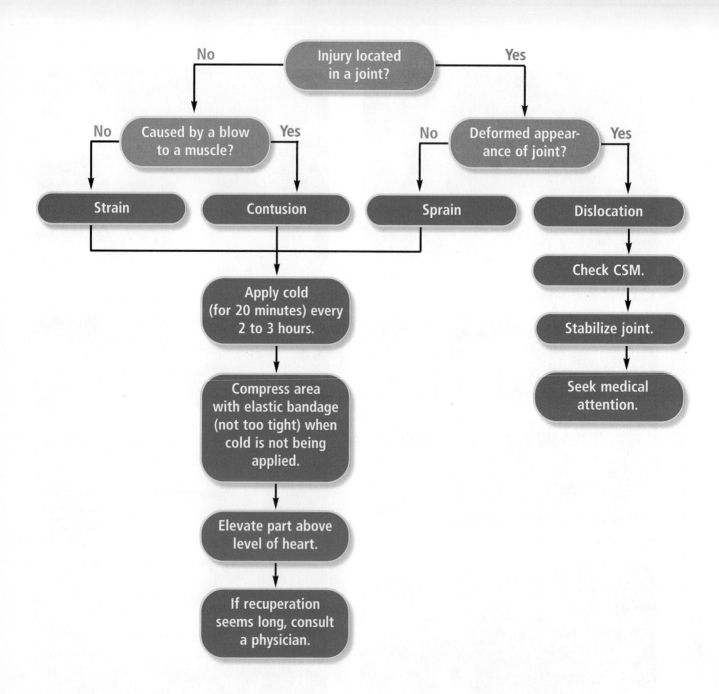

Contusions

A muscle contusion or bruise results from a blow to the muscle.

What to Look For

Any of the following signs and symptoms may occur in a muscle contusion:

- swelling
- pain and tenderness
- black-and-blue mark appearing hours later

What to Do

Use the RICE procedures.

Cramps

A cramp occurs when a muscle goes into an uncontrolled spasm and contraction, resulting in severe pain and restriction or loss of movement.

What to Do

There are many treatments for cramps. Try one or more of the following:

1. Have the victim gently stretch the affected muscle. Because a muscle cramp is an uncontrolled muscle contraction or spasm, a gradual lengthening of the muscle may help lengthen the muscle fibers and relieve the cramp.
2. Relax the muscle by applying pressure to it.
3. Apply ice to the cramped muscle to make it relax, unless you are in a cold environment.
4. Pinch the upper lip hard (an acupressure technique) to reduce calf-muscle cramping.
5. Drink lightly salted cool water (dissolve $\frac{1}{4}$ teaspoon salt in a quart of water) or a commercial sports drink.

Caution:

DO NOT give salt tablets to a person with muscle cramps. They can cause stomach irritation, nausea, and vomiting.

DO NOT massage or rub the affected muscle. This only causes more pain and does not relieve the cramping.

RICE Procedure for Bone, Joint, and Muscle Injuries

RICE is the acronym for the first aid procedures—rest, ice, compression, elevation—for bone, joint, and muscle injuries. The steps you take in the first 48 to 72 hours after such an injury can help to relieve, and even prevent, aches and pains. **Treat all extremity bone, joint, and muscle injuries with the RICE procedures. In addition to RICE, fractures and dislocations should be splinted to stabilize the injured area. (See Chapter 12 for splinting techniques.)**

R = Rest

Injuries heal faster if rested. Rest means the victim stays off the injured part. Using any part of the body increases the blood circulation to that area, which can cause more swelling of an injured part. Crutches may be used to rest leg injuries.

I = Ice

An ice pack should be applied to the injured area for 20 to 30 minutes every two or three hours during the first 24 to 48 hours. Skin treated with cold passes through four stages: cold, burning, aching, and numbness. When the skin becomes numb, usually in 20 to 30 minutes, remove the ice pack. After removing the ice pack, compress the injured part with an elastic bandage and keep it elevated (the "C" and "E" of RICE).

Cold constricts the blood vessels to and in the injured area, which helps reduce the swelling and inflammation as it dulls the pain and relieves muscle spasms. Cold should be applied as soon as possible after the injury—healing time often is directly related to the amount of swelling that occurs. Heat has the opposite effect when applied to fresh injuries: it increases circulation to the area and greatly increases both the swelling and the pain.

Use either of the following methods to apply cold to an injury:

- Put crushed ice (or cubes) into a double plastic bag, hot water bottle. Place the ice pack on the skin and then use an elastic bandage to hold the ice pack in place. Ice bags can conform to the body's contours.
- Use a chemical cold pack, a sealed pouch that contains two chemical envelopes. Squeezing the pack mixes the chemicals, producing a chemical reaction

Skill Scan

RICE Procedures for an Ankle

1

R = Rest
Stop using the injured part. Continued use could cause further injury, delay healing, increase pain, and stimulate bleeding. Get the victim into a comfortable position, either sitting or lying down. This slows blood flow to the injured area.

1. R = Rest

Place ice pack on area.

2. I = Ice

Use elastic bandage to hold ice pack (20 min.).

3. I = Ice

Remove ice pack. Place "U" shaped cloth around ankle knob.

4. C = Compression

Use elastic bandage to hold "U" shaped cloth (3-4 hours).

5. C = Compression

Cover heel and close to the toes.

6. C = Compression

7

E = Elevation
Elevating the injured part is another way to decrease swelling and pain. As you apply ice or compression, elevate the part in a convenient manner. The aim of this step is to get the injured part higher than the heart, if possible.

7. E = Elevation

Repeat cycles of:
• ice pack for 20 minutes followed by
• compression for 3–4 hours for 24 to 48 hours (if severe, 72 hours)

that has a cooling effect. Although they do not cool as well as other methods, they are convenient to use when ice is not readily available. They lose their cooling power quickly, however, and can be used only once. Also, they may be impractical because they are expensive and can break.

Caution:

DO NOT apply an ice pack for more than 20 to 30 minutes at a time. Frostbite or nerve damage can result.

DO NOT apply cold if the victim has a history of circulatory disease, Raynaud's syndrome (spasms in the arteries of the extremities that reduce circulation), abnormal sensitivity to cold, or if the injured part has been frostbitten previously.

DO NOT stop using an ice pack too soon. A common mistake is the early use of heat, which will result in swelling and pain. Use an ice pack three to four times a day for the first 24 hours, preferably up to 48 hours, before applying any heat. For severe injuries, using ice for up to 72 hours is recommended.

C = Compression

Compressing the injured area may squeeze some fluid and debris out of the injury site. Compression limits the ability of the skin and of other tissues to expand and reduces internal bleeding. Apply an elastic bandage to the injured area, especially the foot, ankle, knee, thigh, hand, or elbow. Fill the hollow areas with padding such as a sock or washcloth before applying the elastic bandage.

Elastic bandages come in various sizes, for different body areas:

- 2-inch width, used for the wrist and hand
- 3-inch width, used for the ankle, elbow and arm
- 4- or 6-inch width, used for the ankle, knee, and leg

Start the elastic bandage several inches below the injury and wrap in an upward, overlapping (about one-half the bandage's width) spiral, starting with an even, slightly tight pressure. Gradually wrap more loosely above the injury. Stretch a new elastic bandage to about one third its maximum length for adequate compression. Leave fingers and toes exposed so possible color change can be easily observed. Compare the toes or fingers of the injured extremity with the uninjured one. Pale skin, pain, numbness, and tingling are signs that the bandage is too tight. If any of these symptoms appear, immediately remove the elastic bandage. Leave the elastic bandage off until all the symptoms disappear, then rewrap the area, less tightly. Always wrap from below the injury and move toward the heart.

Applying compression may be the most important step in preventing swelling. The victim should wear the elastic bandage continuously for the first 18 to 24 hours (except when cold is being applied). At night, have the victim loosen but not remove the elastic bandage.

For an ankle injury, place a horseshoe-shaped pad around the ankle knob and secure with the elastic bandage. The pad will help compress the soft tissues rather than just the bones. Wrap the bandage tightest nearest the toes and loosest above the ankle. It should be tight enough to decrease swelling but not tight enough to inhibit blood flow.

For a contusion or a strain, place a pad between the injury and the elastic bandage.

E = Elevation

Gravity slows the return of blood to the heart from the lower parts of the body. Once fluids get to the hands or feet, they have nowhere else to go and those parts of the body swell. Elevating the injured area, in combination with ice and compression, limits circulation to that area, helps limit internal bleeding, and minimizes swelling.

It is simple to prop up an injured leg or arm to limit bleeding. Whenever possible, elevate the injured part above the level of the heart for the first 24 hours after an injury. If a fracture is suspected, do not elevate an extremity until it has been stabilized with a splint. Even then, some fractures should not be elevated.

Along with RICE, fractures and dislocations should be splinted. Chapter 12 describes splinting techniques for various parts of the body.

Caution:

DO NOT apply an elastic bandage too tightly. If applied too tightly, elastic bandages will restrict circulation.

ANKLE INJURIES

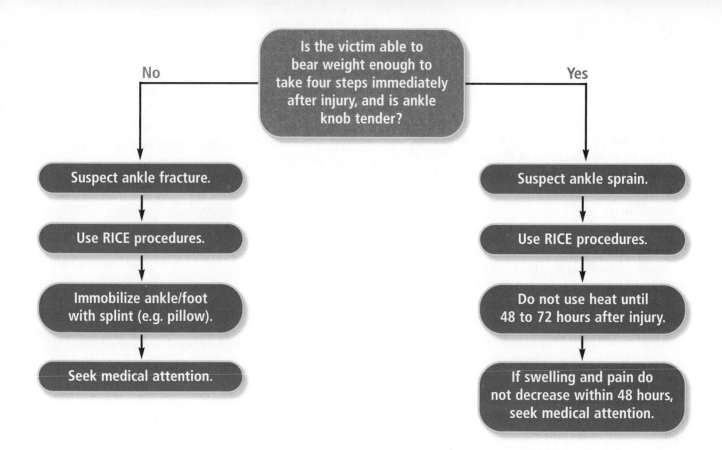

Is the victim able to bear weight enough to take four steps immediately after injury, and is ankle knob tender?

No

Yes

Suspect ankle fracture.

Use RICE procedures.

Immobilize ankle/foot with splint (e.g. pillow).

Seek medical attention.

Suspect ankle sprain.

Use RICE procedures.

Do not use heat until 48 to 72 hours after injury.

If swelling and pain do not decrease within 48 hours, seek medical attention.

Blood under a Nail

When a fingernail has been crushed, blood collects under the nail. This condition usually is very painful because of the pressure of the blood pressing against the nail ▼Figure 4 .

What to Do

1. Immerse the finger in ice water or apply an ice pack with the hand elevated.

2. By using one of the following methods, relieve the pressure under the injured nail:

   - Straighten the end of a metal (noncoated) paper clip or use the blunt (eye) end of a sewing needle. Hold the paper clip or needle with pliers and use a match or cigarette lighter to heat it until the metal is red hot. Press the glowing end of the paper clip or needle against the nail until it melts through. Little pressure is needed. The nail has no nerves, so this is a painless procedure ▶Figure 5 .

   - Using a rotary action, drill through the nail with the sharp point of a knife.

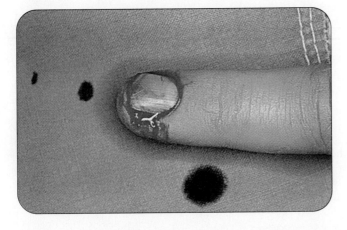

Figure 4 Relieve pain by releasing blood under a nail.

Red-hot, noncoated metal paper clip

Press hot end so it melts through

Figure 5 Making a hole in a fingernail

3. Apply a dressing to absorb the draining blood and to protect the injured nail.

Ring Strangulation

Sometimes a finger is so swollen that a ring cannot be removed. Ring strangulation can be a serious problem if it cuts off circulation long enough. Try one or more of the following methods to remove a ring:

- Lubricate the finger with grease, oil, butter, petroleum jelly, or some other slippery substance, and then try to remove the ring.

- Immerse the finger in cold water or apply an ice pack for several minutes to reduce the swelling.

- Massage the finger from the tip to the hand to move the swelling; lubricate the finger again and try removing the ring.

- Call 9-1-1 or your local emergency number. They can use a ring-cutter to remove the ring when all else fails.

Meeting OSHA Guidelines

This chapter covers the following OSHA Guidelines for First Aid training:

- Section IV. A. 6a-e. Principles and first aid intervention for injuries involving open fractures, closed fractures, and splinting; dislocations, especially the methods of joint dislocations of the upper extremity; joint sprains; muscle strains, contusions, and cramps; and head, neck, back, and spinal injuries.

- Section IV. A. 7a. Proper care for finger and toe nail hematoma, lacerations, splinters, finger avulsion, ring removal, and foreign bodies.

Learning Activities

Fractures

Directions: Circle Yes if you agree with the statement, and circle No if you disagree.

Yes   No   **1.** For a suspected arm or leg fracture, check blood flow and nerves.

Yes   No   **2.** Apply cold on a suspected fracture.

Yes   No   **3.** A splint can help stabilize (keep in place) a fracture.

Scenario: While changing a light bulb in a high ceiling lighting fixture, an electrician falls off a 10-foot ladder. The victim complains about a pain in his left leg. You check the left leg and find some deformity, tenderness, and swelling. What should you do?

_____

_____

_____

Dislocations and Sprains

Yes   No   **1.** The letters RICE represent the treatment for sprains and dislocations.

Yes   No   **2.** When using ice, place it directly on the skin.

Yes   No   **3.** Applying heat too soon to the injury is a common mistake.

Yes   No   **4.** An elastic bandage, if used correctly, can help control swelling in a joint.

Scenario: Your husband comes home limping and in pain. He says he twisted his ankle at work. One of his co-workers told him that it was best to "walk it out." What should you do?

_____

_____

_____

Muscle Injuries

Yes   No   **1.** Give salt tablets to a person suffering muscle cramps.

Yes   No   **2.** Apply heat initially to a muscle injury.

Yes   No   **3.** An elastic bandage, if used correctly, can help limit swelling.

Scenario: During a company softball game, a batter loses her grip while swinging at a pitch. The bat flies through the air and hits a nearby player hard on the thigh. Although the skin is not broken, there is tenderness and some swelling. What should you do?

_____

_____

_____

Chapter 12

Splinting Extremities

Most extremity fractures are minor. Because medical help is usually nearby, the injury can be stabilized by splinting the extremity in the position in which it was found. To stabilize means to use any method to hold a body part still and prevent movement. Before a victim is moved, all fractures should be stabilized to:

- reduce pain
- prevent damage to muscle, nerves, and blood vessels
- prevent a closed fracture from becoming an open fracture
- reduce bleeding and swelling

Types of Splints

A splint is any device used to stabilize a fracture or a dislocation. Such a device can be improvised from a folded newspaper, for example, or it can be a commercial splints (eg, SAM Splint™). Lack of a commercial splint should never prevent you from properly stabilizing an injured extremity ▶Skill Scans.

Splinting sometimes requires improvisation. Improvised splints can be made from folded newspapers, magzines, heavy cardboard, wood, a pillow, a folded blanket, a baseball bat, or an umbrella.

A rigid splint is an inflexible device attached to an extremity to maintain stability. It may be a padded board, a piece of heavy cardboard, or a SAM Splint™ to fit the extremity. Whatever its construction, a rigid splint must be long enough so that it can be secured well above and below the fracture site. A soft splint, such as an air splint, is useful mainly for stabilizing fractures of the lower leg or the forearm.

A self, or anatomic, splint is almost always available. A self splint is one in which the injured body part is tied to an uninjured part. For example, an injured finger can be tied to an adjacent finger, the legs can be tied together, or an injured arm can be tied to the chest.

Splinting Guidelines

All fractures and dislocations should be stabilized before the victim is moved. When in doubt, apply a splint.

Caution:

DO NOT straighten dislocations or fractures of the spine, elbow, wrist, hip, or knee because of the proximity of major nerves and arteries. Instead, if the CSM (circulation-sensation-movement) is all right, splint joint injuries in the position found.

What to Do

1. Cover all open wounds, if any, with a dry, sterile dressing before applying a splint.

2. Check CSM in the extremity. If the pulses are absent, and medical help is hours away, gently straighten a fracture or dislocations to restore blood flow. Straighten the extremity by supporting the limb and moving gently to line up the parts. Do **not** force anything into position. Any movement of a fracture is expected to cause pain and you should be aware of this and warn the patient. You do not have to make the limbs perfectly aligned, just enough to allow the return of circulation.

3. As a general rule, a splint should extend to stabilize the joints above and below the area of the broken bone. For example, stabilize the wrist and elbow for a fractured radius or ulna (bone in the lower arm); stabilize both shoulder and elbow for a fractured humerus (upper arm bone); stabilize both knee and ankle for a fractured tibia or fibula (lower leg bones). An upper extremity fracture, in addition to being splinted, should be placed in an arm sling and a swathe (binder).

4. If two first aiders are present, one should support the injury site and minimize movement of the extremity until splinting is completed.

5. When possible, place splint materials on both sides of the injured part, especially when two bones are involved such as the lower arm's radius and ulna or the lower leg's tibia and fibula. This "sandwich splint" prevents the injured extremity from rotating and keeps the two bones from touching. With rigid splints, use extra padding in natural body hollows and around any deformities.

6. Apply splints firmly but not so tightly that blood flow into an extremity is affected. Check CSM before and after the splint is applied. If the pulse disappears, loosen the splint enough so you can feel the pulse. Leave the fingers or toes exposed so CSM can be checked easily.

7. Use RICE on the injured part. When practical, elevating the injured extremity after stabilization promotes gravity-induced drainage from the limb and reduces swelling. *Do not, however, apply ice packs if a pulse is absent.*

Most fractures do not require rapid transportation. An exception is an arm or a leg without a pulse, which means there is insufficient blood flow to that extremity. In that case, *immediate* medical attention is necessary.

Meeting OSHA Guidelines

This chapter covers the following OSHA Guidelines for First Aid training:

- Section IV. E. 2. Principles and performance of splinting of the arm, elbow, clavicle, fingers, hand, forearm, ribs, hip, femur, lower leg, ankle, knee, foot, and toes.

Skill Scan   Splinting—Upper Extremities

Arm Sling: Shoulder and Clavicle Injuries

Arm Sling and Swathe for Upper Extremity Injuries

Upper Arm (Humerus)

Forearm (Radius/Ulna)

Fingers and Hand (Position of Function)

Skill Scan Splinting—Elbow and Knee

Elbow in Bent Position

Knee in Bent Position

Elbow in Straight Position

Knee in Straight Position

Skill Scan Splinting—Lower Extremities

Lower Leg (Tibia/Fibula)—Rigid Splint

Thigh (Femur)—Rigid Splint

Soft Splint: Ankle/Foot

Self-Splint: Leg

Self-Splint: Fingers/Toes

Learning Activities

Splinting the Extremities

Directions: Circle Yes if you agree with the statement, and circle No if you disagree.

Yes   No   **1.** A splint is a device that can be used to help stabilize a fractured bone.

Yes   No   **2.** A padded board is a type of self-splint.

Yes   No   **3.** When splinting, you should check circulation before and after applying the splint.

Yes   No   **4.** You should attempt to straighten all extremity fractures.

Yes   No   **5.** Splints should only be placed on one side of injured area to maintain adequate circulation.

Yes   No   **6.** Splints should be applied snugly enough to reduce circulation.

Yes   No   **7.** Extremity fractures rarely need more advanced medical attention.

Yes   No   **8.** Splints should extend beyond the joints above and below the injured area.

Scenario: A home builder has fallen from a ladder and possibly broken his wrist. What should you do?

_____

_____

_____

Chapter 13

Sudden Illnesses

Heart Attack

A heart attack happens when the blood supply to part of the heart muscle is severely reduced or stopped. Usually that happens when one of the coronary arteries (the arteries that supply blood to the heart muscle) is blocked by an obstruction or a spasm.

What to Look For

Heart attacks are difficult to determine. Because medical care at the onset of a heart attack is vital to survival and the quality of recovery, if you suspect a heart attack for any reason, seek medical attention *at once*.

Possible signs and symptoms of a heart attack include:

- uncomfortable pressure, fullness, squeezing, or pain in the center of the chest that lasts more than a few minutes or that goes away and comes back
- pain spreading to the shoulders, neck, or arms
- chest discomfort with lightheadedness, fainting, sweating, nausea, or shortness of breath

Not all these warning signs occur in every heart attack. It is difficult to determine if someone is having a heart attack. Many victims will deny that they are experiencing something as serious as a heart attack. Delay can seriously increase the risk of major damage. Insist on taking prompt action.

What to Do

1. Call EMS or get to the nearest hospital emergency department with 24-hour emergency cardiac care.
2. Monitor victim's condition.
3. Help the victim to the least painful position, usually sitting with legs up and bent at the knees ▶Figure 1 . Loosen clothing around the neck and midriff. Be calm and reassuring.
4. Determine if the victim is known to have coronary heart disease and is using nitroglycerin. Nitroglycerin tablets or spray under the tongue or

Half-sitting position.

Support back.

Knees bent.

Place padding under knees.

Figure 1 Help the victim into a relaxed position to ease strain on heart.

nitroglycerin ointment on the skin may relieve chest pain. Nitroglycerin dilates the coronary arteries, which increases blood flow to the heart muscle, and lowers blood pressure and dilates the veins, which decreases the work of the heart and the heart muscle's need for oxygen.

Caution: Because nitroglycerin lowers blood pressure, the victim should sit or lie down once it is taken.

5. If the victim is unresponsive, check ABCs and start CPR, if needed.

Angina

Chest pain called angina pectoris can result from coronary heart disease just as a heart attack does. Angina happens when the heart muscle does not get as much blood as it needs (which means a lack of oxygen).

Angina is brought on by physical exertion, exposure to cold, emotional stress, or the ingestion of food. It seldom lasts longer than 10 minutes and almost always is relieved by nitroglycerin. (In contrast, chest pain from a heart attack is as likely to happen at rest as during activity; the pain lasts longer than 10 minutes and is not relieved by nitroglycerin.)

Stroke (Brain Attack)

A stroke, also referred to as a brain attack or cerebrovascular accident (CVA), occurs when blood vessels that deliver oxygen-rich blood to the brain rupture or become plugged, so part of the brain does not get the blood flow it needs (▼Figure 2). Deprived of oxygen, nerve cells in the affected area of the brain cannot function and die within minutes. Because dead brain cells are not replaced, the devastating effects of a stroke often are permanent.

Transient ischemic attacks (TIAs) are closely associated with strokes. Because TIAs have many of the same signs and symptoms, they often are confused with strokes. The main difference between a TIA and a stroke is that the symptoms of TIA are transient, lasting from several minutes (75% last less than five minutes) to several hours, with a return to normal neurologic function. TIAs are "mini-strokes." A TIA should be considered a serious warning sign of a potential stroke—about one third of all TIA cases will suffer a stroke within 2 to 5 years after their first TIA. Any signs and symptoms of a TIA should be reported to a physician.

What to Look For

- weakness, numbness, or paralysis of the face, an arm, or a leg on one side of the body
- blurred or decreased vision, especially in one eye
- problems speaking or understanding
- dizziness or loss of balance
- sudden, severe, and unexplained headache
- deviation of the pupils of the eyes from PEARL (**P**upils **E**qual **A**nd **R**eactive to **L**ight), which may mean the brain is being affected by lack of oxygen

What to Do

First aid for a stroke victim is limited to supportive care:

1. If victim is unresponsive, check the ABCs.
2. Call EMS.

Figure 2 Severe brain hemorrhage causing a stroke

3. If the victim does not have any injury (from a fall), lay the victim down with the head and shoulders slightly elevated to reduce blood pressure on the brain. Place a victim who is unresponsive but breathing in the recovery position, which is on the side (to keep the airway open and to permit secretions and vomit to drain from the mouth).

Caution:

DO NOT give a stroke victim anything to drink or eat. The throat may be paralyzed, which restricts swallowing.

Asthma
What to Look For

- coughing
- cyanosis (bluish skin color)
- inability to speak in complete sentences without pausing for breath
- nostrils flaring with each breath
- difficulty breathing including wheezing (high-pitched whistling sound during breathing)

What to Do

1. Keep the victim in a comfortable upright position that makes it easier to breathe.
2. Monitor the ABCs.
3. Ask the victim about any asthma medication he or she may be using (▶Figure 3). Most asthma suffer-

ers will have some form of asthma medication, usually administered through physician-prescribed, hand-held inhalers.

4. If the victim does not respond well to his or her inhaled medication or is having an extreme asthma attack (known as status asthmaticus), seek medical attention immediately.

Hyperventilation

Fast, deep breathing is common during emotional stress.

What to Look For

- dizziness or lightheadedness
- numbness
- tingling of the hands and feet
- shortness of breath
- breathing rates faster than 40/min

What to Do

1. Calm and reassure the victim.
2. Encourage the victim to breathe slowly, using the abdominal muscles. Inhale through the nose; hold the full inhalation for several seconds; then exhale slowly. Do NOT have the victim breathe into a paper bag.

Fainting

Most fainting is associated with decreased blood flow to the brain. The decreased blood flow may be caused by low blood sugar (hypoglycemia), slow heart rate (vagal reaction, in which the vagus nerve, which slows the heart rate, is overstimulated by fright, anxiety, drugs, or fatigue), heart-rhythm disturbances, dehydration, heat exhaustion, anemia, or bleeding.

Sitting or standing for a long time without moving, especially in a hot environment, can cause blood to pool in dilated vessels. That results in a loss of effective circulating blood volume, and blood pressure drops. As the blood flow to the brain decreases, the person loses consciousness and collapses.

What to Do

1. Check ABCs.
2. If the victim is unresponsive, but breathing, place the victim in the recovery position.

Asthma medication for an attack.

Keep victim sitting up.

Figure 3 Taking asthma medication

3. Loosen tight clothing and belts.

4. If the victim has fallen, check for any sign of injury. After recovery, have the victim sit for a while. When he or she is able to swallow, give cool, sweetened liquids to drink, and help the victim slowly regain an upright posture.

5. Fresh air and a cold, wet cloth for the face usually aid recovery.

Most fainting episodes are not serious, and the victim recovers quickly. Seek medical attention, however, if the victim

- has had repeated attacks of unconsciousness.
- does not quickly regain consciousness.
- loses consciousness while sitting or lying down.
- faints for no apparent reason.

Seizures

A seizure is the result of an abnormal stimulation of the brain's cells. A variety of medical conditions increase the instability or irritability of the brain and can lead to seizures, including the following:

- epilepsy
- heatstroke
- poisoning
- electric shock
- hypoglycemia
- high fever in children
- brain injury, tumor, or stroke
- alcohol withdrawal, drug abuse/overdose

Epilepsy is not a mental illness, and it is not a sign of low intelligence. It also is not contagious. Between seizures, a person with epilepsy functions normally.

What to Do

The Epilepsy Foundation lists the following first aid procedures for seizures:

1. Cushion the victim's head (a rolled towel or jacket works well); remove items that could cause injury if the person bumped into them.

2. Loosen any tight clothing, especially around the neck.

3. Roll the victim onto his or her side.

4. As the seizure ends, offer your help. Most seizures in people with epilepsy are not medical emergencies.

They end after a minute or two without harm and usually do not require medical attention.

5. Call EMS if any of the following exists:

- A seizure happens to someone who is not known to have epilepsy (eg, there is no "epilepsy" or "seizure disorder" identification). It could be a sign of serious illness.
- A seizure lasts more than five minutes.
- The victim is slow to recover, has a second seizure, or has difficulty breathing afterward.
- The victim is pregnant or has another medical condition.
- There are any signs of injury or illnesses.

Diabetic Emergencies

Diabetes is a condition in which insulin, a hormone produced by the pancreas that helps the body use the energy in food, is either lacking or ineffective (▼**Figure 4**). Insulin is needed to take sugar from the blood and carry it into the cells to be used. If the sugar remains in the blood, the body cells must rely on fat as fuel. Blood sugar (glucose) is a major body fuel, and when it cannot be used, it builds up in the blood, overflows into the urine, and passes out of the body unused so the body loses an important source of fuel. Diabetes develops. Diabetes is not contagious.

Figure 4 Diabetic emergencies

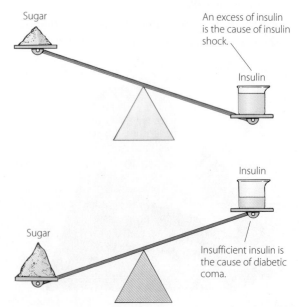

There are two types of diabetes:

- *Type I: juvenile-onset or insulin-dependent* diabetes. Type I diabetics require external (not made by the body) insulin to allow sugar to pass from the blood into cells. When deprived of external insulin, the diabetic becomes quite ill.

- *Type II: adult-onset or non-insulin-dependent* diabetes. Type II diabetics tend to be overweight. They are not dependent on external insulin to allow sugar into cells. However, if their insulin level is low, the lack of sugar in the cells increases sugar production and sugar in the blood to very high levels. That causes glucose to spill into the urine, drawing fluid with it and resulting in dehydration.

The body is continuously balancing sugar and insulin. Too much insulin and not enough sugar leads to low blood sugar, possibly insulin shock. Too much sugar and not enough insulin leads to high blood sugar, possibly diabetic coma.

Low Blood Sugar

Very low blood sugar, called hypoglycemia, is sometimes referred to as an "insulin reaction." This condition can be caused by too much insulin, too little or delayed food, exercise, alcohol, or any combination of these factors.

The American Diabetes Association lists the following signs and symptoms of insulin reaction and hypoglycemia as diabetic emergencies requiring first aid:

- sudden onset
- staggering, poor coordination
- anger, bad temper
- pale color
- confusion, disorientation
- sudden hunger
- excessive sweating
- trembling
- eventual unconsciousness

What to Do

Use the "Rule of 15s" for giving sugar if the victim is a known diabetic, mental status is changed, and is awake to swallow:

1. Give 15 grams of sugar (eg, 2 large teaspoons or lumps of sugar, or one half can of regular soda, or 4 oz. of orange juice, or two to five glucose tablets, or one tube of glucose gel) ▸Figure 5 .

Figure 5 Glucose tablets and gel

2. Wait 15 minutes.
3. If no improvement, give 15 more grams of sugar (carbohydrate).
4. If no improvement, seek immediate medical attention.

High Blood Sugar

Hyperglycemia—also known as diabetic coma—is the opposite of hypoglycemia. Hyperglycemia occurs when the body has too much sugar in the blood. This condition may be caused by insufficient insulin, overeating, inactivity, illness, stress, or a combination of these factors.

The American Diabetes Association lists the following signs and symptoms of diabetic coma and hyperglycemia as diabetic emergencies requiring first aid:

- gradual onset
- drowsiness
- extreme thirst
- very frequent urination
- flushed skin
- vomiting
- fruity breath odor
- heavy breathing
- eventual unconsciousness

What to Do

1. If you are uncertain whether victim has high or low blood-sugar level, give the person food or drink containing sugar.

2. If you do not see improvement in 15 minutes, seek medical care.

DIABETIC EMERGENCIES

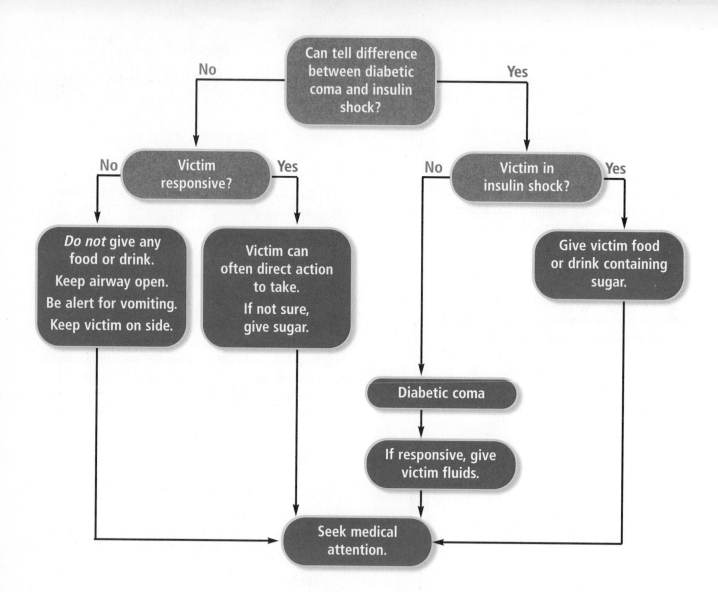

Emergencies During Pregnancy

Most pregnancies are normal and occur without complications. However, sometimes problems do arise and medical attention is required. It is essential that you remain calm, focused, and considerate of the mother during this unforeseen and stressful situation.

What to Look For

Immediately notify a doctor to report the following signs and symptoms in a pregnant woman:

- vaginal bleeding
- cramps in lower abdomen
- swelling of the face or fingers
- severe continuous headache
- dizziness or fainting
- blurring of vision or seeing spots
- uncontrollable vomiting

What to Do

If the victim is experiencing vaginal bleeding or abdominal pain:

1. Keep quiet, warm, and on her left side
2. Have victim or another woman place a sanitary napkin or any sterile or clean pad over the opening of the vagina.
3. Have victim or another woman replace but save any blood-soaked pads and all tissues that are passed. Send this with the woman to medical help for examination by the physician.
4. Arrange for immediate transportation to a medical facility.

If the victim has injuries to her lower abdomen:

1. Keep the woman quiet, warm, and on her left side.
2. Monitor ABCs.
3. Arrange for immediate transportation to a medical facility.

Meeting OSHA Guidelines

This chapter covers the following OSHA Guidelines for First Aid training:

- Section IV. A. 1c. Appropriate assessment and first aid treatment of a victim who has fainted.
- Section IV. A. 8a-f. Principles and first aid intervention for heart attack, stroke, asthma attack, diabetic emergencies, seizures, and pregnancy including the appropriate care of any abdominal injury or vaginal bleeding.

Learning Activities

Sudden Illnesses

Directions: Circle Yes if you agree with the statement, and circle No if you disagree.

Yes No **1.** Heart attack victims experience the least amount of chest pain when lying down.

Yes No **2.** When taking doctor-prescribed nitroglycerin for chest pain, the person should be sitting or lying down.

Yes No **3.** A stroke victim should have his or her head slightly raised.

Yes No **4.** Most asthma victims will usually have a physician-prescribed inhaler.

Yes No **5.** A victim who is breathing fast (hyperventilation) should be encouraged to breathe slowly by holding inhaled air for several seconds, then exhaling slowly.

Yes No **6.** Splash or sprinkle water on a person who has fainted.

Yes No **7.** Have a fainted victim inhale smelling salts or ammonia inhalants.

Yes No **8.** Place a strong stick or similar object between a seizure victim's teeth.

Yes No **9.** A person having seizures always requires medical attention.

Yes No **10.** If in doubt about whether a victim is having an insulin reaction or is in a diabetic coma, give sugar to a responsive victim who can swallow.

Yes No **11.** During a diabetic emergency, if you do not see improvement in 15 minutes, seek medical attention for the victim.

Scenario #1: A 50-year-old co-worker complains about chest pain. He says that it started about an hour ago and has not let up. He is sure that it is just a little indigestion and feels silly about talking about it. He says the pain feels like "something pressing on my chest," and he feels nauseous. What should you do?

_____

_____

Scenario #2: You are working in an office cubicle next to a co-worker who suddenly collapses. You rush to help and find him confused, with numbness and paralysis on one side. Another co-worker says that he earlier complained of a severe headache. What should you do?

_____

_____

Scenario #3: During a first aid training video showing a bloodied victim, a young man suddenly falls from his chair to the floor. He is breathing and has a pulse, but is unresponsive. No other injuries from the fall are detected. What should you do?

_____

_____

Scenario #4: You see some of your co-workers holding down another employee on the floor. They are trying to force a couple of pencils between her teeth. The person is unresponsive and is having severe muscle jerks. What should you do?

_____

_____

Scenario #5: After work, the car-pool driver is driving fast and erratically. When she stops to let her first rider out, she just sits in the car staring ahead. She then slumps over onto the steering wheel. Her skin is cold and sweaty. You are aware the driver is diabetic. What should you do?

_____

_____

Chapter 14

Poisoning

Ingested (Swallowed) Poisons

Fortunately, most poisons ingested have low toxicity or are swallowed in amounts so small that severe poisoning rarely occurs. However, the potential for severe or fatal poisoning is always present.

What to Look For

- abdominal pain and cramping
- nausea or vomiting
- diarrhea
- burns, odor, stains around and in mouth
- drowsiness or unconsciousness
- poison containers nearby

What to Do

1. Determine critical information:
   - Age and size of the victim?
   - What was swallowed? (Read container label; save vomit for analysis.)
   - How much was swallowed (eg, a "taste," half a bottle, a dozen tablets)?
   - When was it swallowed?

2. If a corrosive or caustic (ie, acid or alkali) substance was swallowed, immediately dilute it by having the victim drink at least one or two eight-ounce glasses of water or milk. (*Cold* milk or water tends to absorb heat better than room-temperature or warmer liquids.)

3. *For a responsive victim,* call a poison control center *immediately.* Some poisons do not cause harm until hours later, while others do damage immediately. More than 75% of poisonings can be treated by following the instructions given over the telephone from a poison control center. The center also will advise you if medical attention is needed. Poison control centers routinely follow up calls to check whether additional symptoms or unexpected effects are occurring. The inside front covers of telephone directories contain the number for local poison control centers.

SWALLOWED POISON

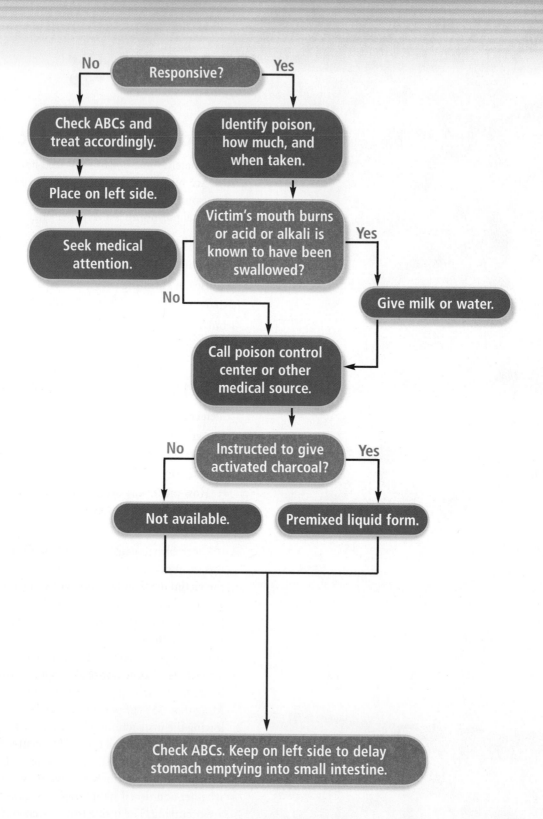

Material Safety Data Sheets (MSDS)

✚ For each hazardous chemical in the workplace, an employer is required by law to maintain a copy of the MSDS. An MSDS lists the hazardous ingredients of a product, its physical and chemical characteristics (eg, flammability), its effects on human health, the chemicals with which it can adversely react, handling precautions, measures that can be used to control exposure, emergency and first aid procedures, and methods to contain a spill.

Figure 2
Activated charcoal

4. *For an unresponsive victim,* check ABCs and treat accordingly. Call 9-1-1 or the local emergency number. Monitor ABCs often.

5. Place the victim on his or her *left* side. This positions the end of the stomach where it enters the small intestine (pylorus) straight up. In this position, gravity will delay (by as much as two hours) the poison's advance into the small intestine, where absorption into the victim's circulatory system is faster **▼Figure 1**. The side position also helps prevent breathing foreign materials into the lungs if vomiting begins. Do not induce vomiting.

6. Give activated charcoal if a poison control center advises **▶Figure 2**. It is the single most effective agent for most swallowed poisons. Activated charcoal acts like a sponge to bind and keep the poison in the digestive system, thus preventing its absorption into the blood.

   Although activated charcoal may appear similar to burnt-toast scrapings and charcoal briquettes, these items *cannot* be used for poisoning.

   Not all chemicals, however, are absorbed well by activated charcoal, including acids and alkalis (eg, bleach, ammonia), potassium, iron, alcohol, methanol, kerosene, cyanide, malathion, and ferrous sulfate.

   A drawback of activated charcoal is its grittiness and its appearance. Trying to improve the taste or consistency by adding chocolate syrup, sherbet, ice cream, milk, or other flavoring agents only decreases the charcoal's binding capacity. Place the charcoal mixture in an opaque container and have the victim sip it through a straw so it will be more palatable. First aiders should give only the pre-mixed form. Some common names for the pre-mixed form are Actidose™, InstaChar™, and LiquiChar™

   Although activated charcoal is an inexpensive, safe, and effective means for decreasing poison absorption, pharmacies do not routinely stock it.

7. Save poison containers, plants, and the victim's vomit to help medical personnel identify the poison.

Caution:

DO NOT give water or milk to dilute poisons unless instructed to do so by a poison control center. Fluids may dissolve a dry poison (eg, tablets or capsules) more rapidly and fill up the stomach, forcing stomach contents (ie, the poison) into the small intestine, where poisons are absorbed faster.

Alcohol and Other Drug Emergencies
Alcohol Intoxication

Helping an intoxicated person is often difficult since the individual may be belligerent and combative. Also, per-

Figure 1 The left-side position delays the poison from advancing into the small intestine.

Place on left side

Position for poisoned victim

sonal hygiene is sometimes less than optimal. However, it is important that alcohol abusers be helped and not just labeled as "drunks." Their condition may be quite serious, even life-threatening.

What to Look For

Although the following signs indicate alcohol intoxication, some may also mean illness or injury other than alcohol abuse, such as diabetes or heat injury:

- the odor of alcohol on a person's breath or clothing
- unsteady, staggering walking
- slurred speech and the inability to carry on a conversation
- nausea and vomiting
- flushed face

Caution:

DO NOT let an intoxicated person sleep on his or her back.

DO NOT leave an intoxicated person alone.

DO NOT try to handle a hostile intoxicated person by yourself. Find a safe place, then call the police for help.

What to Do

First aid for an intoxicated person includes these steps:

1. Look for any injuries. Alcohol can mask pain.
2. Check ABCs and treat accordingly.
3. If the intoxicated person is lying down, place him or her in the recovery position. Rolling the victim onto the left side not only reduces the likelihood of vomiting and aspiration of vomit, but also delays absorption of alcohol into the bloodstream.
4. Call the poison control center for advice or the local emergency number for help.
5. Provide emotional support, but if the victim becomes violent, leave the scene and find a safe place until police arrive.
6. If the intoxicated victim has been exposed to the cold, suspect hypothermia and move the person to a warm environment whenever possible. Remove wet clothing and cover the individual with warm blankets. Handle a hypothermic victim gently, because rough handling could induce a heart attack.

Drugs Other Than Alcohol

What to Do

1. Check ABCs.
2. Call the poison control center for advice or EMS for help.
3. Check for injuries.
4. Keep the person on the *left* side to reduce the likelihood of vomiting and aspiration of vomit and to delay the absorption of drugs into the bloodstream.
5. Provide reassurance and emotional support.
6. If the person becomes violent, find a safe place until the police arrive. Let law enforcement officers handle dangerous situations.
   What to look for:
   • drowsiness, anxiety, or agitation
   • dilated or large pupils
   • confusion
   • hallucinations
   • rapid heart rate

Carbon Monoxide Poisoning

Carbon monoxide (CO) victims are often unaware of its presence. The gas is invisible, tasteless, odorless, and non-irritating. It is produced by the incomplete burning of organic material such as gasoline, wood, paper, charcoal, coal, and natural gas.

What to Look For

It is difficult to tell if a person is a CO victim.
   The following conditions indicate possible CO poisoning:

- The symptoms come and go.
- The symptoms worsen or improve in certain places or at certain times of the day.
- People around the victim have similar symptoms.
- Pets seem ill.

The signs and symptoms of CO poisoning are as follows:
- headache
- ringing in the ears (tinnitus)
- chest pain (angina)
- muscle weakness
- nausea and vomiting
- dizziness and visual changes (blurred or double vision)
- unconsciousness
- respiratory and cardiac arrest

What to Do

1. Get the victim out of the toxic environment and into fresh air *immediately.*
2. Call EMS personnel, who will be able to give the victim 100% oxygen, improving oxygenation.
3. Monitor ABCs.
4. Place an unresponsive victim in the recovery position.
5. Seek medical attention. All suspected CO victims should obtain a blood test to determine the level of CO.

Plant-Induced Dermatitis: Poison Ivy, Poison Oak, and Poison Sumac

Most people cannot identify these irritating plants (▼Figure 3A–B). A helpful method of identifying these plants is the "black-spot test." When the sap is exposed to the air, it turns brown in a matter of minutes and by the next day is black.

Figure 3A Poison ivy, found in all 48 contiguous states in the U.S.

Figure 3B Poison ivy dermatitis

What to Do

1. Those who know they have been in contact with a poisonous plant should decontaminate the skin as soon as possible (within five minutes for sensitive people, up to one hour for moderately sensitive individuals). Use soap and cold water to clean the skin of the oily resin or apply rubbing (isopropyl) alcohol liberally (not in swab-type dabs). If too little isopropyl alcohol is used, the oil will actually spread to another site and enlarge the injury. Rinse with water to remove the solubilized material. Water removes the urushiol (plant resin) from the skin, oxidizes and inactivates it, and does not penetrate the skin as do solvents. Unfortunately, most victims do not know about their contact until several hours or days later, when the itching and rash begin.

2. If the reaction is mild, the person can soak in a lukewarm bath sprinkled with one to two cups of colloidal oatmeal, such as Aveeno™ Colloidal oatmeal, or apply any of the following:
   - calamine lotion (calamine ointment if the skin becomes dry and cracked) or zinc oxide
   - baking soda paste: one teaspoon of water mixed with three teaspoons of baking soda

3. If the reaction is mild to moderate, care for the skin as you would for a mild reaction and use a physician-prescribed corticosteroid ointment. Oral antihistamines such as Benadryl™ often are used in conjunction with prescription creams to help decrease itching.

4. For a severe reaction, follow the same care guidelines for the skin and use a physician-prescribed oral corticosteroid (eg, prednisone). Apply a topical corticosteroid ointment or cream.

Meeting OSHA Guidelines

This chapter covers the following OSHA Guidelines for First Aid training:

- Section IV. A. 3a. Principles and first aid intervention for alkali, acid and systemic poisons; know how and when to contact the local Poison Control Center.
- Section IV. A. 3b. Principles and first aid intervention for inhaled poisons, importance of assessing the toxic potential of the environment to the rescuer and the need for respirators, the acute effect of chemicals utilized in worksites, the location of chemical inventories, material safety data sheets (MSDS's), chemical emergency information, and antidote supplies.
- Section IV. A. 3c. Principles and first aid intervention for topical poisons including poison ivy, poison sumac, poison oak, and insecticides.
- Section IV. A. 3d. Principles and first aid intervention for drugs of abuse including alcohol, narcotics, tranquilizers, and amphetamines.

Learning Activities

Poisoning

Directions: Circle Yes if you agree with the statement, and circle No if you disagree.

Yes   No   **1.** If a corrosive or caustic substance was swallowed, you may dilute it by having the victim drink water or milk.

Yes   No   **2.** For a poisoned victim, call a poison control center immediately.

Yes   No   **3.** Use activated charcoal if advised by poison control.

Yes   No   **4.** Place a swallowed poison victim on his or her left side to delay the poison from going into the small intestine.

Yes   No   **5.** Do NOT let an intoxicated person sleep on his or her back.

Yes   No   **6.** If an intoxicated or drugged person becomes violent, leave the scene and let law enforcement officers handle the situation.

Yes   No   **7.** Seek medical attention for all carbon monoxide victims.

Yes   No   **8.** Calamine lotion can help relieve itching caused by poison ivy, oak, or sumac.

Yes   No   **9.** Some cases of poison ivy, oak, or sumac require medical attention.

Scenario #1: You find your two-year-old son, Scott, vomiting. You notice the top of a nearby medicine container is off. The label on the container indicates that the medicine belongs to your mother who is visiting. You realize that Scott must have swallowed some of the highly potent medicine. What should you do?

_____

_____

Scenario #2: At a party given by your boss, one of the guests becomes quite drunk. He vomits and is now unresponsive. What should you do?

_____

_____

Scenario #3: A 25-year-old co-worker seems to be "freaking out." Another co-worker says she saw the victim take some "pills." After she finally calms down, she tells you that she took some drugs. What should you do?

_____

_____

Scenario #4: A driver is waiting in his truck until the building workers can load it. He's left the motor running to keep the heater on and has closed all the windows and doors because of the subfreezing outside temperatures. When the building workers come to tell him they're ready, he is slumped over the wheel. They move him to fresh air just as you arrive. What should you do?

_____

_____

Scenario #5: While weeding around a vacant lot, you pull up a batch of weeds with shiny leaves in clusters of three. You finish the job about an hour later. The next morning your arms are itching, and you notice a rash beginning to appear. What should you do?

_____

_____

Chapter 15

Bites and Stings

Animal Bites

It is estimated that one of every two Americans will be bitten at some time by an animal or by another person. As it is commonly interpreted, the term animal bite in this section refers to a bite by a mammal, not by an insect or reptile. Dogs are responsible for about 80% of all animal-bite injuries (▶Figure 1).

Rabies

A virus found in warm-blooded animals causes rabies. The disease spreads from one animal to another in the saliva, usually through a bite or by licking.

Consider an animal as possibly rabid if any of the following applies:

- The animal attacked without provocation.
- The animal acted strangely, that is, out of character (eg, a usually friendly dog is aggressive, or a wild fox seems docile and "friendly").
- The animal was a high-risk species (skunk, raccoon, or bat).

What to Do

1. If the victim was bitten in the United States (except for the area along the border with Mexico) by a healthy domestic dog or cat, the animal will likely be confined and observed for 10 days for any illness. If necessary, a veterinarian will kill the animal (domesticated or wild), decapitate it, and send the head to a laboratory for analysis. If the animal is dead when you find it, transport the entire body; do not attempt decapitation (precautions must be taken to prevent exposure to potentially infected tissues and saliva).

   Report animal bites to the police or animal control officers; they should be the ones to capture the animal for observation. If the dog or cat escapes and is not suspected to be rabid, consult local public health officials.

Figure 1 Dog bite

If the victim was bitten in the United States by a skunk, raccoon, bat, fox, or other mammal, it should be considered a rabies exposure and treatment should be started *immediately*. The only exception is when the bite occurred in a part of the continental United States known to be free of rabies. If the wild animal is captured, it should be killed and its head shipped to a qualified laboratory immediately.

2. Clean the wound with a soap solution and rinse it with water under pressure.

3. Stop the bleeding and give wound care.

4. Seek medical attention for further wound cleaning and a possible tetanus shot. The physician will determine if sutures are needed to close the wound. If needed, a vaccination series against rabies will be started.

Human Bites

The human mouth contains a wide range of bacteria, so the chance of infection is greater from a human bite than from bites of other warm-blooded animals.

What to Do

1. If the wound is not bleeding heavily, wash it with soap and water (under the pressure from a faucet) for 5 to 10 minutes. Avoid scrubbing, which can bruise tissues.

2. Rinse the wound thoroughly with running water under pressure.

3. Control bleeding with direct pressure.

4. Cover the wound with a sterile dressing. Do *not* close the wound with tape or butterfly bandages, which traps bacteria in the wound and increases the chance of infection.

5. Seek medical attention for possible further wound cleaning, a tetanus shot, and sutures to close the wound (if needed).

Snakebites

Only four snake species in the United States are venomous: rattlesnakes (which account for about 65% of all venomous snakebites and nearly all the snakebite deaths in the United States), copperheads, water moccasins (also known as cottonmouths), and coral snakes (▼Figure 2). The first three are pit vipers. The coral snake is small and colorful, with a black snout and a series of bright red, yellow, and black bands around its body (every other band is yellow).

Pit Viper Bites
What to Look For

- severe burning pain at the bite site
- two small puncture wounds about 1/2 inch apart (some cases may have only one fang mark) (►Figure 3)
- swelling (happens within five minutes and can involve an entire extremity)
- discoloration and blood-filled blisters possibly developing in 6 to 10 hours (►Figure 4)

Figure 2 Rattlesnake

Figure 3 Rattlesnake bite (Note two fang marks)

Figure 4 Copperhead bite two hours after bite

- in severe cases, nausea, vomiting, sweating, and weakness

In about 25% of poisonous snakebites, there is no venom injection, only fang and tooth wounds (known as a "dry" bite).

What to Do

Identifying the type of pit viper is of minimal importance, because the same antivenin is used in all cases in North America.

The Wilderness Medical Society lists the following guidelines for dealing with bites by pit vipers:

1. Get the victim and bystanders away from the snake. Snakes have been known to bite more than once. Pit vipers can strike as far away as one half of their body length. Be careful around a decapitated snake head—head reactions can persist for 20 minutes or more.

2. Do not attempt to capture or kill the snake. It wastes valuable time, there is a risk of additional bites, and identification of the snake is not usually needed since the same antivenin is used for all pit viper bites.

3. Keep the victim quiet. If possible, carry the victim or have the victim walk very slowly to help minimize exertion.

4. Gently wash the bitten area with soap and water. Any ring(s) or jewelry that might reduce blood circulation if swelling occurs should be removed.

5. Stabilize the bitten extremity (arm or leg) with a sling or a splint as you would for a fracture. Keep the extremity below heart level despite the fact that swelling may occur..

6. Seek medical attention *immediately.* This is the most important thing to do for the victim. Antivenin must be given within four hours of the bite (not every venomous snakebite requires antivenin).

Coral Snake Bites

The coral snake is America's most venomous snake, but it rarely bites people. The coral snake has short fangs and tends to hang on and "chew" its venom into the victim rather than to strike and release, like a pit viper.

What to Do

1. Keep the victim calm.
2. Gently clean the bite site with soap and water.

3. Apply mild pressure by wrapping an elastic bandage (eg, Ace™ bandage) over the bite site and the entire arm or leg. You should apply pressure only if the bite is from a coral snake, not any of the pit vipers. Do *not* cut the victim's skin or use a Sawyer Extractor™.

4. Seek medical attention for antivenin.

Nonpoisonous Snakebites

A nonpoisonous snake leaves a horseshoe shape of toothmarks on the victim's skin. If you are not positive about a snake, assume it was venomous. Some so-called nonpoisonous North American snakes such as hognose and garter snakes have venom that can cause painful local reactions but no systemic (whole-body) symptoms.

What to Do

1. Gently clean the bite site with soap and water.
2. Care for the bite as you would a minor wound.
3. Seek medical advice.

Insect Stings

Severe allergic reactions to insect stings are reported by about 0.5% of the population in the United States. Fortunately, localized pain, itching, and swelling—the most common consequences of an insect bite—can be treated with first aid.

What to Look For

A rule of thumb is that the sooner symptoms develop after a sting, the more serious the reaction will be.

What to Do

Most people who have been stung can be treated on site, and everyone should know what to do if a life-threatening allergic reaction (anaphylaxis) occurs. In particular, those who have had a severe reaction to an insect sting should be instructed on what they can do to protect themselves. They also should be advised to wear a medical-alert identification tag stating they are insect allergic.

1. Check the sting site to see if a stinger and venom sac are embedded in the skin. Bees are the only stinging insects that leave their stingers and venom sacs behind (▶Figure 6). If the stinger is still embedded, remove it or it will continue to inject poison for two or three minutes. Scrape the stinger and venom sac

Figure 6 Honeybee

away with a hard object such as a long fingernail, credit card, scissor edge, or knife blade. If applied in the first three minutes, a Sawyer Extractor™ can remove a portion of the venom.

2. Wash the sting site with soap and water to prevent infection.

3. Apply an ice pack over the sting site to slow absorption of the venom and relieve pain. Because bee venom is acidic, a paste made of baking soda and water can help. Sodium bicarbonate is an alkalinizing agent that draws out fluid and reduces itching and swelling.

    Wasp venom, on the other hand, is alkaline, so apply vinegar or lemon juice.

4. To further relieve pain and itching, some type of pain medication usually is adequate. A topical steroid cream, such as hydrocortisone, can help combat local swelling and itching. An antihistamine may prevent some local symptoms and later reactions if given early, but it works too slowly to counteract a life-threatening allergic reaction.

5. Observe the victim for at least 30 minutes for signs of an allergic reaction. Epinephrine is an effective treatment for a person with a severe allergic reaction. A person with a known allergy to insect stings should have a physician-prescribed emergency kit that includes prefilled syringes of epinephrine. Because epinephrine is short-acting, watch the victim closely for signs of returning anaphylaxis. Inject another dose of epinephrine as often as every 15 minutes if needed, available, and consistent with the directions for use in the kit.

Spider Bites

Most spiders are venomous, which is how they paralyze and kill their prey. But spiders lack an effective delivery system (long fangs and strong jaws) to bite a human. Death occurs rarely and only from bites by brown recluse and black widow spiders.

A spider bite is difficult to diagnose, especially when the spider was not seen or recovered, because the bites typically cause little immediate pain.

Black Widow Spiders

Black widow spiders have round abdomens that vary in color from gray to brown to black, depending on the species (▼Figure 7). In the female black widow, the abdomen is shiny black with a red or yellow spot (often in the shape of an hourglass) or white spots or bands. Black widow spiders are found throughout the world.

What to Look For

It is difficult to determine if a person has been bitten by a black widow spider or, for that matter, by any spider.

- The victim may feel a sharp pinprick when the spider bites, but some victims are not even aware of the bite. Within 15 minutes, a dull, numbing pain develops in the bite area.

Figure 7 Black widow spider. Note red hourglass configuration on abdomen.

- Two small fang marks might be seen as tiny red spots.
- Within 15 minutes to four hours, muscle stiffness and cramps occur, usually affecting the abdomen when the bite is on a lower part of the body and the shoulders, back, or chest when the bite is on an upper part. Victims often describe the pain as the most severe they have ever experienced.
- Headache, chills, fever, heavy sweating, dizziness, nausea, and vomiting appear next. Severe pain around the bite site peaks in two to three hours and can last 12 to 48 hours.

Brown Recluse Spiders

Brown recluse spiders are also known in North America as fiddle-back or violin spiders (▶Figure 8A). They have a violin-shaped figure on their backs (several other spider species have a similar configuration on their backs). Color varies from fawn to dark brown, with darker legs.

Brown recluse spiders are found primarily in the southern and midwestern states, with other, less toxic, related spiders throughout the rest of the country. They are absent from the Pacific Northwest where the aggressive house spider, also known as the hobo spider, is found and causes injuries similar to those of the brown recluse.

What to Look For

- A local reaction usually occurs within two to eight hours with mild to severe pain at the bite site and redness, swelling, and local itching.
- In 48 to 72 hours, a blister develops at the bite site, becomes red, and bursts. During the early stages, the affected area often takes on a bull's-eye appearance, with a central white area surrounded by a reddened area, ringed by a whitish or blue border (▶Figure 8B). A small, red crater remains, over which a scab forms. When that scab falls away in a few days, a larger crater remains. That also scabs over and falls off, leaving a yet larger crater. The craters are known as *volcano lesions.* This process of slow tissue destruction can continue for weeks or even months. The ulcer sometimes requires skin grafting.
- Fever, weakness, vomiting, joint pain, and a rash may occur.
- Stomach cramps, nausea, and vomiting may occur.

Tarantulas

Tarantulas bite only when vigorously provoked or roughly handled. The bite varies from almost painless to a deep throbbing pain lasting up to 1 hour. The tarantula, when upset, will roughly scratch the lower surface of its abdomen with its legs and flick hairs onto the invader's skin. The hairs cause itching and hives that can last several weeks. Treatment is cortisone cream and antihistamines.

What to Do (for All Spider Bites)

1. If possible, catch the spider to confirm its identity. Even if the body has been crushed, save it for identification (although most spider-bite victims never see the spider). The species helps determine the treatment, so the dead spider (if it can be found) should be taken with the victim to the hospital.

2. Clean the bite area with soap and water or rubbing alcohol.

3. Place an ice pack over the bite to relieve pain and delay the effects of the venom.

4. Monitor ABC.

5. Seek medical attention immediately. An antivenin exists for black widow spider bites. It is usually reserved for children (under 6 years), the elderly (over 60 and with high blood pressure), pregnant women, and victims with severe reactions. The antivenin will give relief within 1 to 3 hours. Antivenin for brown recluse and other spider bites is not currently available.

Figure 8A Brown recluse spider. Note violin or fiddle configuration on back.

Figure 8B Brown recluse spider bite. Note bull's-eye approach.

Scorpion Stings

Scorpions look like miniature lobsters, with lobster-like pincers and a long upcurved "tail" with a poisonous stinger (▼Figure 9). Several species of scorpions inhabit the southwestern United States, but only the bark scorpion poses a threat to humans.

What to Look For

The most frequent symptom of a scorpion sting, especially in an adult victim, is local, immediate pain and burning around the sting site. Later, numbness or tingling occurs.

Figure 9 Scorpion

What to Do

1. Monitor ABCs.
2. Gently clean the sting site with soap and water or rubbing alcohol.
3. Apply an ice pack over the sting site.
4. Seek medical attention. Small children are prime candidates for receiving antivenin. An antivenin is available only in Arizona.

Embedded Ticks

Removing Ticks

Remove ticks as soon as possible. If a tick is carrying a disease, the longer it stays embedded, the greater the chance of the disease being transmitted.

Because its bite is painless, a tick can remain embedded for days without the victim's realizing it (▼Figure 10). Most tick bites are harmless, although ticks can carry serious diseases.

Figure 10 Deer ticks: not engorged and blood engorged

1. To pull a tick off (▼Figure 11),
   - Use tweezers or one of the specialized tick-removal tools. Grasp the tick as close to the skin as possible and lift the tick with enough force to "tent" the skin surface. Hold in this position until the tick lets go. This may take several seconds. Do not pull hard enough to break the tick apart, as this will leave parts of the tick behind that will cause infection.
2. Wash the bite site with soap and water. Apply rubbing alcohol to further disinfect the area.
3. Apply an ice pack to reduce pain.
4. Apply calamine lotion to relieve any itching. Keep the area clean.
5. Continue to watch the bite site for one month for a rash. If a rash appears, see a physician. Watch for other signs such as fever, muscle aches, sensitivity to bright light, and paralysis that begins with leg weakness.

Figure 11 Removing a tick with tweezers

Meeting OSHA Guidelines

This chapter covers the following OSHA Guidelines for First Aid training:

- Section IV. A. 7a. Principles and first aid intervention for human and animal (especially dog and snake) bites.
- Section IV. A. 7b. Principles and first aid intervention for bites and stings from insects (spiders, ticks, scorpions, hornets, and wasps), including responses to anaphylactic shock; other allergic manifestations; and rabies and tetanus prophylaxis.

Learning Activities

Bites and Stings

Directions: Circle Yes if you agree with the statement, and circle No if you disagree.

Yes No   **1.** Report animal bites to the police or animal control officers.

Yes No   **2.** Apply cold or ice over a snakebite.

Yes No   **3.** Use the "cut-and-suck" method for a snakebite.

Yes No   **4.** Snakes have been known to bite more than once.

Yes No   **5.** Apply a cold or ice pack over an insect sting or a suspected spider bite.

Yes No   **6.** A baking soda paste can help reduce the itching and swelling from an insect sting.

Yes No   **7.** A victim's doctor-prescribed epinephrine injector may have to be given if the victim has a life-threatening reaction to an insect sting.

Yes No   **8.** Spider bite antivenin is available for only black widow spider bites, and not all victims need it.

Yes No   **9.** A capsule with antihistamine or cortisone ointment or tablet can be useful for mosquito bites.

Yes No   **10.** Applying a blown-out, glowing match head or heated needle will cause an embedded tick to back out of a victim's skin.

Yes No   **11.** Cover an embedded tick with heavy oil or grease to make the tick back out because of lack of oxygen.

Scenario #1: A mail carrier is heard crying for help while being attacked by a neighbor's large dog. The dog's owner calls off the dog and takes it inside his house. You run up the street and help the victim over to a nearby yard. You find several severe bite marks on the mail carrier's legs and arms. What should you do?

_____

_____

Scenario #2: You rush to a vacant lot to help a young woman who is calling for help. She says that some type of snake bit her on the leg. You see two puncture wounds (fang marks) on her leg. What should you do?

_____

_____

Scenario #3: A garden shop employee complains about her face swelling and a feeling of tightness across her chest. She is having some breathing difficulty. She says a bee stung her. She has a medical alert tag around her neck indicating an allergy to insects. She tells you that she has medication for such an emergency. There is an ice machine nearby. What should you do?

_____

_____

Scenario #4: While resting during lunch in the patio behind your office building, you feel a sharp pinprick on your arm. About 15 minutes later, a dull, numbing pain develops in your back. You look at your arm and see two tiny red spots. About an hour later, abdominal cramping starts and steadily gets worse. What should you do?

_____

_____

Scenario #5: On a Monday morning, one of your co-workers returns from a weekend camping trip. When he rubs the back of his head, he feels a bump and asks you to look at it. You see a tick embedded in his scalp. What should you do?

_____

_____

Chapter 16

Cold-Related Emergencies

Freezing Injuries

Most injuries from cold are confined to exposed areas of the body, such as the face, or to extremities such as the fingers and toes (▶Figures 1–3). Freezing cold injuries can occur whenever the air temperature is below freezing (32°F). Freezing limited to the skin surface is frostnip. Freezing that extends deeper through the skin and into the flesh is frostbite.

Frostnip is caused by water freezing on the skin surface. The skin becomes reddened and possibly swollen. Although frostnip is painful, there usually is no further damage after rewarming. Repeated frostnip in the same spot can dry the skin, causing it to crack and to become sensitive. It is difficult to tell the difference between frostnip and frostbite. Frostnip should be taken seriously because it may be the first sign of impending frostbite. To treat frostnip:

1. Gently warm the affected area by placing it against a warm body part (eg, put bare hands under the armpits or on the stomach or blow warm air on the area).

2. Do not rub the area. After rewarming, the affected area may be red and tingling.

Frostbite occurs when temperatures drop below freezing. Frostbite affects mainly the feet, hands, ears, and nose. These areas do not contain large heat-producing muscles and are some distance from the body's heat-generating sources. The most severe consequences of frostbite are gangrene and amputation.

What to Look For

The exact severity and extent of frostbite are difficult to judge until hours after thawing, although before thawing it can be classified as *superficial* or *deep*. Even physicians have to wait until thawing has occurred before they can judge the extent of the injury.

FROSTBITE

Figure 1 Frostbitten fingers, 6 hours after rewarming in 106° water

Figure 2 Second-degree frostbite

The signs and symptoms of superficial frostbite are:

- Skin color is white, waxy, or grayish-yellow.
- The affected part feels very cold and numb. There may be tingling, stinging, or aching sensations.
- The skin surface feels stiff or crusty and the underlying tissue feels soft when depressed gently and firmly.

Deep frostbite is indicated by the following signs and symptoms:

- The affected part feels cold, hard, and solid and cannot be depressed.
- The affected part is cold, with pale, waxy skin.
- A painfully cold part suddenly stops hurting.
- Blisters may appear after rewarming.

After a part has thawed, frostbite can be categorized by degrees, similar to the burn classifications.

What to Do

Frostbite injuries require the following first aid treatment.

1. Get the victim out of the cold and into a warm place.
2. Remove any clothing or constricting items that could impair blood circulation (eg, rings).
3. Seek immediate medical attention.
4. Place dry, sterile gauze between toes and the fingers to absorb moisture and to keep them from sticking together.
5. Slightly elevate the affected part to reduce pain and swelling.

Figure 3 Frostbitten ear 8 hours old

If the victim is in a remote or wilderness situation (more than 1 hour from a medical facility), and you have warm water, use the following wet, rapid rewarming method.

1. Place the frostbitten part in warm (102°F to 105°F) water. If you do not have a thermometer, pour some of the water over the inside of your arm or put your elbow into it to test that it is warm, not hot. Maintain water temperature by adding warm water as needed. Rewarming usually takes 20 to 40 minutes or until the tissues are soft. For ear or facial injuries, apply warm moist cloths, changing them frequently.
2. After thawing,
   - Treat victim as a "stretcher" case—the feet will be impossible to use after they are rewarmed.

- Protect the affected area from contact with clothing and bedding.

- Place dry, sterile gauze between the toes and the fingers to absorb moisture and to keep them from sticking together.

- Slightly elevate the affected part to reduce pain and swelling.

- Apply aloe vera gel to promote skin healing.

- Give the victim ibuprofen to limit pain and inflammation.

Hypothermia

Body temperature falls when the body cannot produce heat as fast as it is being lost. Hypothermia is a life-threatening condition when the body's core temperature falls below 95°F. Hypothermia does not require subfreezing temperatures.

What to Look For

- *Change in mental status.* This is one of the first symptoms of developing hypothermia. Examples are disorientation, apathy, and changes in personality, such as unusual aggressiveness.

- *Shivering.* Shivering is the first and most important body defense against a falling body temperature. *Shivering* starts when the body temperature drops 1°F *and can produce more heat than many rewarming methods.* As the core temperature continues to fall, however, shivering stops at about 90°F. Shivering also stops as body temperature rises. If shivering stops as responsiveness decreases, assume that the core temperature is falling.

- *Cool abdomen.* Place the back of your hand between the clothing and the victim's abdomen to assess the victim's temperature. When the victim's abdominal skin under clothing is cooler than your hand, consider the victim hypothermic until proved otherwise.

- *Low core body temperature.* The best indicator of hypothermia is a thermometer reading of the core body temperature, but normal thermometers do not register below 94°F, and so do not indicate whether the hypothermia is mild or severe. Rectal temperatures are measured seldom.

Types of Hypothermia

In severe hypothermia, the victim becomes so cold that shivering stops. That means the victim's body cannot rewarm itself internally and will require external heat for recovery.

Victims of mild hypothermia have a core body temperature above 90°F. Symptoms are shivering, slurred speech, memory lapses, and fumbling hands. Victims frequently stumble and stagger, but they are usually responsive and can talk. Mild hypothermia victims will have the "-umbles": grumbles, mumbles, fumbles, and stumbles.

What to Do

1. For all hypothermic victims, stop further heat loss:

   - Get the victim out of the cold.

   - Add insulation such as blankets, towels, pillows, or newspapers beneath and around the victim. Cover the victim's head.

   - Replace wet clothing with dry clothing.

   - Handle the victim gently. Rough handling can cause cardiac arrest.

   - Keep the victim in a horizontal (flat) position.

2. Call EMS.

Adding heat to a victim is extremely difficult. The longer the victim is exposed to the cold, the longer it will take to raise the core temperature to normal. Trying to rewarm a hypothermic victim may cause cardiac arrest.

Although surface rewarming suppresses shivering, it may be the only option when the victim is far from medical care. In that case, the victim must be warmed by any available external heat source.

Meeting OSHA Guidelines

This chapter covers the following OSHA Guidelines for First Aid training:

- Section IV. A. 5a. Principles and first aid intervention for exposure to cold, including frost bite and hypothermia.

HYPOTHERMIA

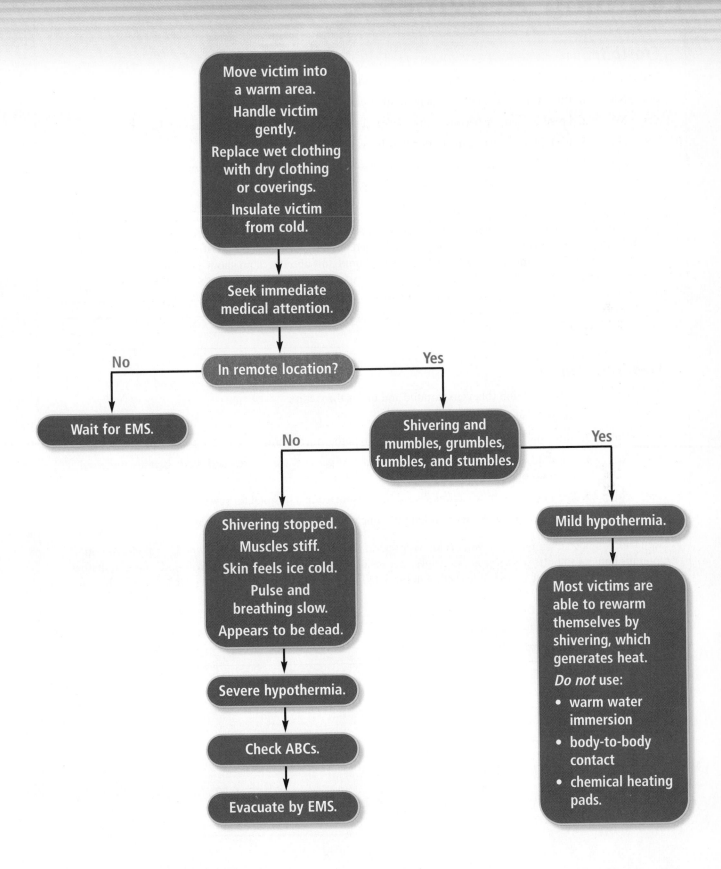

Move victim into a warm area.

Handle victim gently.

Replace wet clothing with dry clothing or coverings.

Insulate victim from cold.

↓

Seek immediate medical attention.

↓

In remote location?

No → Wait for EMS.

Yes → Shivering and mumbles, grumbles, fumbles, and stumbles.

No → Shivering stopped. Muscles stiff. Skin feels ice cold. Pulse and breathing slow. Appears to be dead.

↓

Severe hypothermia.

↓

Check ABCs.

↓

Evacuate by EMS.

Yes → Mild hypothermia.

↓

Most victims are able to rewarm themselves by shivering, which generates heat.

Do not use:
- warm water immersion
- body-to-body contact
- chemical heating pads.

Learning Activities

Frostbite

Directions: Circle Yes if you agree with the statement, and circle No if you disagree.

Yes   No   **1.** Rub or massage to rewarm a frostbitten part.

Yes   No   **2.** Frostbite damage becomes more severe if the affected area thaws and then refreezes.

Yes   No   **3.** It's best to rewarm a frostbitten part by using warm water.

Yes   No   **4.** Placing frostbitten hands in another person's armpits is the best rewarming method.

Yes   No   **5.** When near a hospital, it's best to let medical personnel thaw the frostbitten part.

Scenario: In subfreezing temperatures during a snowstorm, you find a stalled truck on a little-used road. Inside the truck is an elderly man, who tells you that his truck is out of gasoline and that when he tried to refill the truck's gas tank he dropped the gas can and some of the gasoline spilled on his hands. He has been stranded for over 3 hours. The man complains of numb fingers and cold feet. He did not know about a cabin about a quarter mile away. What should you do?

_____

_____

_____

_____

Hypothermia

Yes   No   **1.** Add insulation (blankets) around and under the victim.

Yes   No   **2.** Replace wet clothing with dry clothing.

Yes   No   **3.** Shivering is sufficient to rewarm a mild hypothermic victim.

Yes   No   **4.** For mild hypothermia, applying chemical heat packs or using a rescuer's body heat are preferred methods of rewarming a victim.

Yes   No   **5.** Severe hypothermic victims should be transported to a hospital for rewarming.

Yes   No   **6.** Check the pulse of a severely hypothermic victim for at least 30 to 45 seconds.

Scenario: It is a cold winter day so you decide to check on your 80-year-old grandfather, who lives alone. As you enter his home, you notice that it is not much warmer inside the house than it is outside. You find your grandfather wrapped in a blanket lying on top of his bed. You speak to him, but you get only mumbling. He is severely shivering. What should you do?

_____

_____

_____

_____

Chapter 17

Heat-Related Emergencies

Heat Illnesses

Heat illnesses include a range of disorders. Some of them are common, but only heatstroke is life-threatening. Untreated heatstroke victims always die.

Heat Cramps

Heat cramps are painful muscular spasms that happen suddenly, usually immediately after exertion. They usually involve the muscles in the back of the leg (calf and hamstring muscles) or the abdominal muscles. Some experts claim they are caused by salt depletion. Victims may be drinking fluids that do not have adequate salt content. However, other experts disagree, claiming the typical American diet is heavy with salt.

Heat Exhaustion

Heat exhaustion is characterized by heavy perspiration with normal or slightly above normal body temperatures. It is caused by water or salt depletion or both. Some experts believe that a better term would be severe dehydration. Heat exhaustion affects workers and athletes who do not drink enough fluids while working or exercising in hot environments. Symptoms include severe thirst, fatigue, headache, nausea, vomiting, and sometimes diarrhea. The affected person often mistakenly believes he or she has the flu. Uncontrolled heat exhaustion can evolve into heatstroke.

Heatstroke

Two types of heatstroke exist: classic and exertional. Classic heatstroke, also known as the "slow cooker," may take days to develop. It is often seen during summer heat waves and typically affects the poor, elderly, chronically ill, alcoholic, or obese. Because the elderly, who often have medical problems, are frequently afflicted, this type of

HEAT-RELATED EMERGENCIES

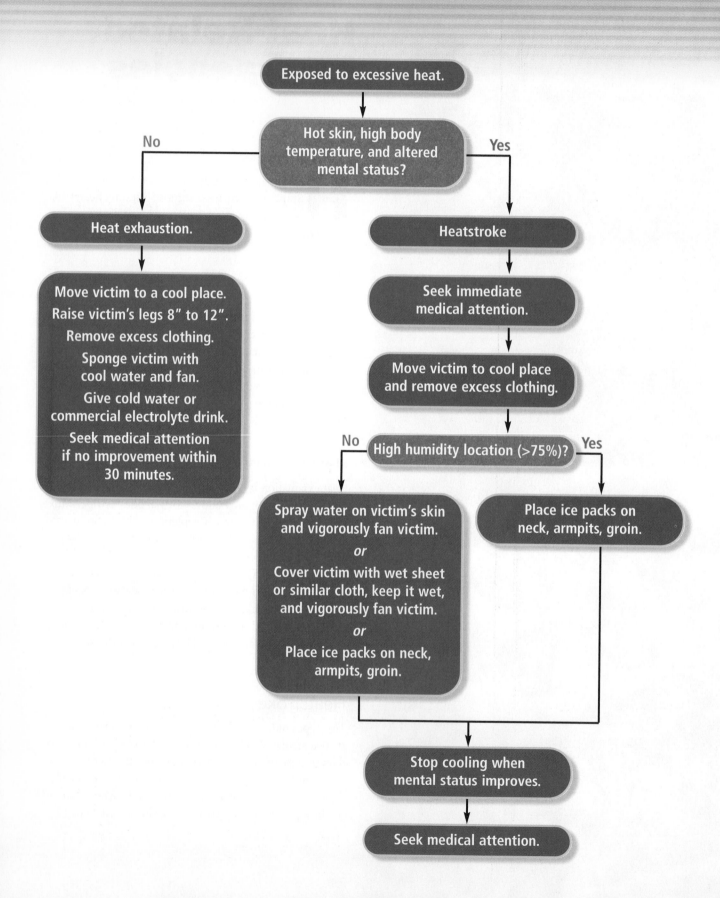

heatstroke has a 50% death rate, even with medical care. It results from a combination of a hot environment and dehydration. Exertional heatstroke is also more common in the summer. It is frequently seen in athletes, laborers, and military personnel, all of whom often sweat profusely. This type of heatstroke is known as the "fast cooker." It affects healthy, active individuals who are strenuously working or playing in a warm environment. Because its rapid onset does not allow enough time for severe dehydration to occur, 50% of exertional heatstroke victims usually are sweating. (Classic heatstroke victims are not sweating.)

There are several ways to tell the difference between heat exhaustion and heatstroke. First, if the victim's body feels extremely hot when touched, suspect heatstroke. Another major mark of heatstroke is altered mental status (behavior), ranging from slight confusion and disorientation to coma. Between those extreme conditions, victims usually become irrational, agitated, or even aggressive and may have seizures. In severe cases, the victim can go into a coma in less than an hour. The longer a coma lasts, the less the chance for survival.

A third way to distinguish heatstroke from heat exhaustion is by rectal temperature. That is not very practical, however, because a responsive heatstroke victim may not cooperate. Taking a rectal temperature can be embarrassing to both victim and rescuer. Moreover, rectal thermometers are seldom available.

What to Do

Heat Cramps

To relieve heat cramps (it may take several hours), follow these steps:

1. Rest in a cool place.
2. Drink lightly salted cool water (dissolve $\frac{1}{4}$ teaspoon salt in a quart of water) or a commercial sports drink.
3. Stretch the cramped calf muscle, or try an acupressure method: pinch the upper lip just below the nose.

Heat Exhaustion

1. Move the victim immediately out of the heat to a cool place.
2. Give cool liquids, adding electrolytes (lightly salted water or a commercial sports drink) if plain water does not improve the victim's condition in 20 minutes. Do not give salt tablets; they can irritate the stomach and cause nausea and vomiting.
3. Raise the victim's legs 8 to 12 inches (keep the legs straight).
4. Remove excess clothing.
5. Sponge with cool water and fan the victim.
6. If you don't see any improvement within 30 minutes, seek medical attention.

Heatstroke

Heatstroke is a medical emergency and must be treated rapidly! Every minute delayed increases the likelihood of serious complications or death.

1. Seek immediate medical attention, even if the victim seems to be recovering.
2. Move the victim immediately to a cool place.
3. Remove all clothing down to the victim's underwear.
4. Keep the victim's head and shoulders slightly elevated.
5. The only way to prevent damage is to cool the victim quickly and by any means possible. Cooling methods include the following:

   - *Spraying* the victim with water and then *fanning*. This method is not as effective in high-humidity (more than 75%) conditions.
   - Apply cool wet sheets or towels.
   - Place ice bags against the large veins in the groin, arm-pits, and sides of the neck to cool the body regardless of the humidity.

Meeting OSHA Guidelines

This chapter covers the following OSHA Guidelines for First Aid training:

- Section IV. A. 5a. Principles and first aid intervention for exposure to heat, including heat cramps, heat exhaustion, and heat stroke.

Learning Activities

Heat-Related Emergencies

Directions: Circle Yes if you agree with the statement, and circle No if you disagree.

Yes   No   **1.** For heat cramps, stretch a cramped leg muscle.

Yes   No   **2.** Salt tablets can be given to victims of any heat illness.

Yes   No   **3.** Move heat illness victims out of the heat to a cool place.

Yes   No   **4.** Heat exhaustion victims need immediate medical attention—it's a life-threatening condition.

Yes   No   **5.** Heatstroke victims need immediate cooling by any means possible.

Yes   No   **6.** Apply rubbing alcohol on a heatstroke victim's skin for cooling.

Yes   No   **7.** If in high-humidity conditions, spray and fan the heatstroke victim.

Yes   No   **8.** In low humidity conditions, only cold or ice packs applied to the neck, armpits, and groin will work well to cool a heatstroke victim.

Scenario #1: A teenager's summer job is mowing lawns for various companies in an industrial park. He is sweating heavily on a very hot, humid day. He complains about being very thirsty, nauseous, and having a headache. What should you do?

_____

_____

_____

Scenario #2: On your vacation, you spend a day at a large amusement park. It is an extremely hot and humid day. During the afternoon, you decide to rest and watch one of the special shows. Soon after you sit down, an elderly man in front of you suddenly falls forward out of his seat. When you reach him, his wife reports that they have been walking around the park practically all day without stopping. His skin feels very hot and dry, and he is unresponsive. What should you do?

_____

_____

_____

Scenario #3: In January, a high-ranking company official from Buffalo has flown to Florida to inspect a new assembly plant. He is accustomed to the cold conditions of the north but not to the heat and humidity of the southeast. He spent the morning inspecting the new plant. Satisfied with what he's seen, he accepts an invitation to golf in the afternoon. While putting at the sixteenth hole, he becomes dizzy and faints, but soon becomes responsive. What should you do?

_____

_____

_____

Chapter 18

Rescuing and Moving Victims

Victim Rescue

Water Rescue

Reach-throw-row-go identifies the sequence for attempting a water rescue. The first and simplest rescue technique is to *reach* for the victim. Reaching requires a lightweight pole, ladder, long stick, or any object that can be extended to the victim. Once you have your "reacher," secure your footing and have a bystander grab your belt or pants for stability. Secure yourself before reaching for the victim.

You can *throw* anything that floats—empty picnic jug, empty fuel or paint can, life jacket, floating cushion, piece of wood, inflated spare wheel—whatever is available. If there is a rope handy, tie it to the object to be thrown so you can pull the victim in, or, if you miss, you can retrieve the object and throw it again. The average untrained rescuer has a throwing range of about 50 feet.

If the victim is out of throwing range and there is a rowboat, canoe, motor boat, or boogie board nearby, you can try to *row* to the victim. Maneuvering these craft requires skills learned through practice. Wear a personal flotation device (PFD) for your own safety. To avoid capsizing, never pull the victim in over the side of a boat; pull over the stern (rear end).

If the reach–throw–row techniques are impossible and you are a capable swimmer trained in water lifesaving procedures, you can *go* to the drowning victim by swimming. Entering even calm water makes a swimming rescue difficult and hazardous. All too often a would-be rescuer becomes a victim as well.

Caution:

DO NOT swim to and grasp a drowning person unless you are trained to make the rescue.

Ice Rescue

If a person has fallen through the ice near the shore, extend a pole or throw a line with a floatable object attached to it. When the person has hold of the object, pull him or her toward the shore or the edge of the ice.

If the person has fallen through the ice away from the shore and you cannot reach him or her with a pole or a throwing line, lie flat and push a ladder, plank, or similar object ahead of you. You can tie a rope to a spare tire and the other end to an anchor point, lie flat, and push the wheel ahead of you. Pull the person ashore or to the edge of the ice.

Caution:

DO NOT go near broken ice without support.

Electrical Emergency Rescue

Electrical injuries can be devastating. Just a mild shock can cause serious internal injuries. A current of 1,000 volts or more is considered high voltage, but even the 110 volts of household current can be deadly.

When a person gets an electric shock, electricity enters the body at the point of contact and travels along the path of least resistance (nerves and blood vessels). The current travels rapidly, generating heat and causing destruction.

Most indoor electrocutions are caused by faulty electrical equipment or careless use of electrical appliances. Before you touch the victim, turn off the electricity at the circuit breaker, fuse box, or outside switch box or unplug the appliance (if the plug is undamaged).

If the electrocution involves high-voltage *power lines,* the power must be turned off before anyone approaches a victim. If you approach a victim and feel a tingling sensation in your legs and lower body, stop. You are on energized ground, and an electrical current is entering one foot, passing through your lower body, and leaving through the other foot. If that happens, raise one foot off the ground, turn around, and hop to a safe place. Wait for trained personnel with the proper equipment to cut the wires or disconnect them.

If a power line has fallen over a car, tell the driver and passengers to stay in the car. A victim should try to jump out of the car *only* if an explosion or fire threatens, and then without making contact with the car or the wire.

Caution:

DO NOT touch an appliance or the victim until the current is off.

DO NOT try to move downed wires.

DO NOT use *any* object, even dry wood (broomstick, tools, chair, stool) to separate the victim from the electrical source.

Hazardous Materials Incidents

At almost any highway crash scene, there is the potential danger of hazardous chemicals. Clues that indicate the presence of hazardous materials include:

- signs on vehicles (eg, "explosive," "flammable," "corrosive")
- spilled liquids or solids
- strong, unusual odors
- clouds of vapor

Stay well away and upwind from the area. Only those who are specially trained in handling hazardous materials and who have the proper equipment should be in the area.

Motor Vehicle Crashes

In most states, you are legally obligated to stop and give help when you are involved in a motor vehicle crash. If you come on a crash shortly after it happens, the law does not require you to stop, although it might be argued that you have a moral responsibility to render any aid you can.

1. Stop and park your vehicle well off the highway or road and out of active traffic lanes. Park at least 5 car lengths from the crash. If the police have taken charge, do not stop unless you are asked to do so. If the police or other emergency vehicles have not arrived, call or send someone to call 9-1-1 or the local emergency number as soon as possible. Ways to call include:
   - Find a pay phone or roadside emergency phone.
   - Use a cellular phone or CB radio.
   - Ask to use a phone at a nearby house or business.

2. Turn on your vehicle's emergency hazard flashers. Raise the hood of your vehicle to draw more attention to the scene.

3. Make sure everyone on the scene is safe.

- Ask the driver(s) to turn off the ignition or turn it off yourself.
- Ask bystanders to stand well off the roadway.
- Place flares or reflectors 250 to 500 feet behind the crash scene to warn oncoming drivers of the crash. Do not ignite flares around leaking gasoline or diesel fuel.

4. If the driver or passenger is unresponsive or might have spinal injuries, use your hands to stabilize their heads and necks.

5. Check and keep monitoring the ABCs. Treat any life-threatening injuries.

6. Whenever possible, wait for EMS personnel to extricate the victims from vehicles, because they have training and the proper equipment. In most cases, keep the victims stabilized inside the vehicle.

7. Allow the EMS ambulance to take victims to the hospital.

Caution:

DO NOT rush to get victims out of a car that has been in a crash. Contrary to opinion, most vehicle crashes do not involve fire, and most vehicles stay in an upright position.

DO NOT move or allow victims to move unless there is an immediate danger like fire or oncoming traffic. Treat victims as though every bone in their bodies is broken.

DO NOT transport victims in your car or any other bystander's vehicle.

Fires

If you encounter a fire, you should:

1. Get all the people out fast.
2. Call the emergency telephone number (usually 9-1-1).

Then—and *only* then—if the fire is small and if your own escape route is clear, should you fight the fire yourself with a fire extinguisher. You may be able to put out the fire or at least hold damage to a minimum.

To use a fire extinguisher, aim directly at whatever is burning and sweep across it. Extinguishers expel their contents quickly, in 8 to 25 seconds for most home models containing dry chemicals.

Caution:

DO NOT get trapped while fighting a fire. Always stay close to an open door so you can exit if the fire gets too big.

Confined Spaces

A confined space is an area not intended for human occupancy that also has the potential for containing or accumulating a dangerous atmosphere. There are three types of confined spaces: below-ground, ground-level, and above-ground. Below-ground confined spaces include manholes, below-ground utility vaults, storage tanks, old mines, cisterns, and wells. Ground-level confined spaces include industrial tanks and farm storage silos. Above-ground confined spaces include water towers and storage tanks.

An accident in a confined space demands immediate action. If someone who enters a confined space signals for help or becomes unconscious, follow these steps to help:

1. Call for immediate help.
2. Do *not* rush in to help.
3. Activate EMS.
4. Do *not* enter the confined space unless you have the proper training and equipment, such as self contained air supply, safety harness, and lifeline.
5. Once the victim is removed, provide care.

Triage: What to Do with Multiple Victims

You may encounter emergency situations in which there are two or more victims. This often happens in multiple-car accidents or disasters. After making a quick scene survey, decide who must be cared for and transported first. This process of prioritizing or classifying injured victims is called "triage." *Triage* is a word taken from the French word "trier," which means *to sort*. The goal is to do the greatest good for the greatest number of victims.

Finding Life-Threatened Victims

A variety of systems are used to identify care and transportation priorities. To find those needing immediate care for life-threatening conditions, first tell all victims who can get up and walk to move to a specific area. Victims who can get up and walk rarely have life-threatening injuries. These victims ("walking wounded") are classified as "delayed priority" (see below). Do not force a victim to move if he or she complains of pain.

Find the life-threatened victims by performing only the initial survey (ABC) on all remaining victims. Go to motionless victims first. You must move quickly (spend less than 60 seconds with each victim) from one victim to the next until all have been assessed. Classify victims according to the following care and transportation priorities:

1. *Immediate care.* Victim has life-threatening injuries but can be saved.

   - airway or breathing difficulties (not breathing or breathing rate slower than 8 per minute or faster than 24 per minute)
   - weak or no pulse
   - uncontrolled or severe bleeding
   - unresponsive or unconscious

2. *Urgent care.* Victims not fitting into the immediate or delayed categories. Care and transportation can be delayed up to one hour.

3. *Delayed care.* Victims with minor injuries. Care and transportation can be delayed up to 3 hours.

4. *Dead.* Victims are obviously dead, mortally wounded, or unlikely to survive because of the extent of their injuries, age, and medical condition.

Do not become involved in treating the victims at this point, but ask knowledgeable bystanders to care for immediate life-threatening problems (ie, rescue breathing, bleeding control).

Reassess victims regularly for changes in their condition. Only after victims with immediate life-threatening conditions receive care should those with less serious conditions be given care.

Later, you will usually be relieved when more highly trained emergency personnel arrive on the scene. You may then be asked to provide first aid, to help move victims, or to help with ambulance or helicopter transportation.

Moving Victims

A victim should not be moved until he or she is ready for transportation to a hospital, if required. All necessary first aid should be provided first. A victim should be moved only if there is an immediate danger (▶Skill Scan):

- There is a fire or danger of fire.
- Explosives or other hazardous materials are involved.
- It is impossible to protect the scene from hazards.
- It is impossible to gain access to other victims in the situation (eg, a vehicle) who need lifesaving care.

A cardiac arrest victim is usually moved unless he or she is already on the ground or floor, because CPR must be performed on a firm surface.

Caution:

DO NOT move a victim unless you absolutely have to, such as when the victim is in immediate danger or must be moved to shelter while waiting for the EMS to arrive.

Emergency Moves

The major danger in moving a victim quickly is the possibility of aggravating a spine injury. In an emergency, every effort should be made to pull the victim in the direction of the long axis of the body to provide as much protection to the spinal cord as possible. If victims are on the floor or ground, you can drag them away from the scene by using various techniques.

Nonemergency Moves

All injured parts should be stabilized before and during moving. If rapid transportation is not needed, it is helpful to practice on another person about the same size as the injured victim.

Meeting OSHA Guidelines

This chapter covers the following OSHA Guidelines for First Aid training:

- Section III. B. 3. The principles of triage.
- Section IV. A. 9a. The danger of entering a confined

space to administer first aid without having the appropriate respiratory protection.

- Section IV. E. 3. Moving and rescuing victims, including one and two person lifts, ankle and shoulder pulls, and the blanket pull.

Skill Scan Drags

1. *Shoulder drag.* For short distances over a rough surface, stabilize victim's head with your forearms.

2. *Ankle drag.* The fastest method for a short distance on a smooth surface.

3. *Blanket pull.* Roll the victim onto a blanket and pull from behind the victim's head.

Skill Scan

One-Person Moves

1. *Human crutch (one person helps victim to walk).* If one leg is injured, help the victim to walk on the good leg while you support the injured side.

2. *Cradle carry.* Use for children and lightweight adults who cannot walk.

3. *Firefighter's carry.* If the victim's injuries permit, you can travel longer distances if you carry the victim over your shoulder.

4. *Pack-strap carry.* When injuries make the fireman's carry unsafe, this method is better for longer distances.

5. *Piggyback carry.* Use this method when the victim cannot walk but can use the arms to hang onto the rescuer.

Skill Scan — Two/Three-Person Moves

1. *Two-person assist.* Similar to human crutch.

2. *Two-handed seat carry.*

3. *Four-handed seat carry.* The easiest two-person carry when no equipment is available, and the victim cannot walk but can use the arms to hang onto the two rescuers.

4. *Extremity carry.*

5. *Chair carry.* Useful for a narrow passage or up or down stairs. Use a sturdy chair that can take the victim's weight.

6. *Hammock carry.* Three to six people stand on alternate sides of the injured person and link hands beneath the victim.

Learning Activities

Rescuing and Moving Victims

Directions: Circle Yes if you agree with the statement, and circle No if you disagree.

Yes   No   **1.** You should attempt to move downed power lines away from a victim, using a broom or other wooden object.

Yes   No   **2.** Strong, unusual odors or clouds of vapor are possible indications of the presence of hazardous materials.

Yes   No   **3.** To keep from getting trapped while attempting to extinguish a fire, you should always keep a door behind you for rapid exit.

Yes   No   **4.** When triaging victims, airway and breathing difficulties are classified as urgent care priorities.

Yes   No   **5.** A major concern in moving a victim quickly is the possibility of aggravating a spine injury.

Yes   No   **6.** "Row – throw – reach – and go" represents the safe order for executing a water rescue.

Yes   No   **7.** In most states, you are not legally obligated to stop and give help when you are involved in a motor vehicle crash.

Scenario: A co-worker has been hurt in an explosion in a lab. He has been thrown across the room and is lying motionless on the floor. You determine it is safe to help, but are afraid there could be another explosion. What should you do?

_____

_____

_____

Appendix A · First Aid Supplies

Workplace First Aid Kit*

Equipment	Minimum Quantity
1. Adhesive strip bandages (1" × 3")	20
2. Triangular bandages (muslin, 36" – 40" × 36" – 40" × 52" – 56")	4
3. Sterile eye pads (2 1/8" × 2 5/8")	2
4. Sterile gauze pads (4" × 4")	6
5. Sterile nonstick pads (3" × 4")	6
6. Sterile trauma pads (5" × 9")	2
7. Sterile trauma pads (8" × 10")	1
8. Sterile conforming roller gauze (2" width)	3 rolls
9. Sterile conforming roller gauze (4 1/2" width)	3 rolls
10. Waterproof tape (1" × 5 yards)	1 roll
11. Porous adhesive tape (2" × 5 yards)	1 roll
12. Elastic roller bandages (4" and 6")	1 each
13. Antiseptic skin wipes, individually wrapped	10
14. Medical-grade exam gloves (medium, large, extra large), conforming to FDA requirements	2 pairs per size
15. Mouth-to-barrier device, either a face mask with a one-way valve or a disposable face shield	1
16. Disposable instant-activating cold packs	2
17. Resealable plastic bags (quart size)	2
18. Padded malleable splint (SAM splint™, 4" × 36")	1
19. Emergency blanket, Mylar	1
20. Paramedic shears (with one serrated edge)	1
21. Splinter tweezers (about 3" long)	1
22. Biohazard waste bag (3 1/2 gallon capacity)	2
23. First aid and CPR manual and list of local emergency telephone numbers	1

* This list does not include over-the-counter ointments, topicals, or internal medicines; consult the workplace's medical director for these.

Gauze rolls   Conforming, self-adhering roller bandages

Medical exam gloves   Face shield   Face mask

Bandage scissors   Tweezers

EMT shears   Regular scissors   Knife

Meeting OSHA Guidelines

This chapter covers the following OSHA Guidelines for First Aid training:

- Section III. G. The first aid provider should be responsible for the type, amount, and maintenance of first aid supplies needed for their particular worksite. These supplies need to be stored in a convenient area available for emergency access.

Appendix B

Automated External Defibrillators (AEDs)

Public Access Defibrillation

Through the implementation of state public access defibrillation (PAD) laws, automated external defibrillators (AEDs) are readily available in many places for trained rescuers to use. These trained rescuers include:

- Firefighters
- EMTs
- Police officers
- Security personnel
- Flight attendants
- Lifeguards
- Office workers
- Lay persons

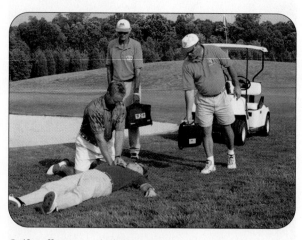

Golf staff arrive to help an apparent heart attack victim.

When Electrical Activity Is Interrupted

Ventricular fibrillation (V-Fib) is the most common abnormal heart rhythm in cases of sudden cardiac arrest in adults.

The organized wave of electrical impulses that causes the heart muscle to contract and relax in a regular fashion is lost when the heart is in ventricular fibrillation. As a result, the lower chambers of the heart quiver and cannot pump blood, so circulation is lost (no pulse).

A second, potentially life-threatening electrical problem is ventricular tachycardia (V-Tach), in which the heart beats too fast to pump blood effectively.

The abnormal heart rhythm known as ventricular fibrillation.

Care for Cardiac Arrest

When the heart stops beating, the blood stops circulating, cutting off all oxygen and nourishment to the entire body. Time is a crucial factor. For every minute that defibrillation is delayed the victim's chance of survival decreases 7 to 10 percent.

Cardiopulmonary resuscitation (CPR) is the initial care for cardiac arrest, until a defibrillator is available.

An automated external defibrillator (AED) is an electronic device that analyzes the heart rhythm and delivers an electrical shock to the heart of a person in cardiac arrest in an effort to reestablish a heart rhythm that will generate a pulse. All AEDs are attached to the victim by a cable connected to two adhesive pads that are placed on the victim's chest. The pad and cable system sends the electrical signal from the heart into the device for analysis and delivers the electric shock to the victim when needed.

The AED analyzes and delivers a shock through two adhesive pads placed on the victim's chest.

AEDs also record the victim's heart rhythm, known as an electrocardiogram (ECG), shock data, and other information about the device performance (e.g., date, time, number of shocks supplied).

AEDs have built-in rhythm analysis systems that determine whether the victim needs a shock. This enables a wide range of people to deliver early defibrillation, with only minimal training required.

There are many different AED models. The principles for use are the same for each, but the displays, controls, and options vary slightly.

a. FirstSave by Cardiac Science
b. LifePak 500 by Medtronic Physio-Control
c. FR2 by Phillips Medical Systems (showing its pediatric pads)

Basic Operation of an AED

If you are going to be using an AED, you must become familiar with the operation of the specific device you will use. The basic operation of all AED models follows this sequence:

1. Turn the power on.
2. Apply the electrode pads to the victim's bare chest.
3. Initiate rhythm analysis.
4. Deliver a shock if indicated.

Read the manufacturer's instructions, which come with the AED, to familiarize yourself with its specific features.

Photo and Illustration Credits

Chapter 1
Opener © Mark E. Gibson; **Figure 1** courtesy of Ellis and Associates

Chapter 2
Opener © Brian Pieters, Masterfile

Chapter 3
Opener © 1998 Bob Winsett/Index Stock Imagery/PictureQuest; **Figures 1 & 4** courtesy of American Academy of Orthopaedic Surgeons (AAOS)

Chapter 4
Opener © Bruce Ayres, Tony Stone

Chapter 5
Opener © 1988 Peter Menzel/Stock, Boston/PictureQuest

Chapter 6
Opener © Christopher Morris/Black Star Publishing/PictureQuest; **Figures 1B, 5** courtesy of AAOS; **Figure 2** © Howard Backer

Chapter 7
Opener © Frank Pedrick/Index Stock Imagery/PictureQuest

Chapter 8
Opener © Owen Franken/Stock, Boston/PictureQuest; **Figure 2** courtesy of AAOS

Chapter 9
Opener © 1992 Tim Lynch/Stock, Boston/PictureQuest

Chapter 10
Opener © Custom Medical Stock Photo

Chapter 11
Opener © 1999 Jim Pickerell/Stock Connection/PictureQuest

Chapter 12
Opener © Custom Medical Stock Photo

Chapter 13
Opener © Wedgworth, Custom Medical Stock Photo; **Figure 5** courtesy of AAOS

Chapter 14
Opener © 1991 Stephen Agricola/Stock, Boston/PictureQuest; **Figure 2** courtesy of AAOS

Chapter 15
Opener © David Dennis, Animals Animals

Chapter 16
Opener © Howard Backer

Chapter 17
Opener © Bob Daemmrich/Stock, Boston/PictureQuest

Chapter 18
Opener © Mark E. Gibson

Appendix B
Figure 1 courtesy of AAOS

Skill Scan

Using an AED

Step 1.

1. Check scene safety.
2. Establish unresponsiveness.
3. Open the airway and check breathing.
4. Administer two slow breaths if victim is not breathing.
5. Check carotid pulse.
6. If second rescuer is available, begin CPR until the AED is applied.

Step 2.

1. Turn power on.
2. Apply electrode pads to victim's chest.
3. Plug in pad connector.

Step 3.

1. Stand clear and analyze.

Step 4.

1. If shock is indicated, clear victim.
2. Press to shock (1st shock).

Step 5.

1. Analyze.
2. If shock is indicated, clear victim.
3. Press to shock (2nd shock).

Skill Scan — Using an AED

Step 6.

1. Analyze.
2. If shock is indicated, clear victim.
3. Press to shock (3rd shock).

Step 7.

1. Check pulse.
2. If no pulse, perform CPR for one minute.
3. Re-analyze.

Step 8.

1. If no pulse, repeat steps 3 through 7.

Step 9.

1. If "No shock indicated" message appears, check pulse.
2. If no pulse, perform CPR for one minute.
3. If no pulse after one minute of CPR, press to analyze.
4. If the victim regains a pulse, follow basic life support procedures.
5. Recheck pulse and breathing; victims successfully defibrillated often return to VF.
6. Follow local protocols for the number of shocks administered prior to arrival of EMS personnel.

Caution:

CHILDREN– For children ages 1-8, use an AED that has been shown to be accurate for this age group. Use child pads, if available.

WATER– Do not use an AED if the victim's chest is wet. A small puddle of water or snow will not impact the use of an AED, as long as the chest is dry.

Automated External Defibrillator Skills Checklist

Student's Name _____ **Date** _____

Skills	Satisfactory	Unsatisfactory
Check for scene safety	○	○
Initial Assessment and Care:		
(If two rescuers are involved, one assesses and performs CPR while the other applies the AED.)		
Establish unresponsiveness	○	○
Have someone call 9-1-1 and get AED	○	○
Open airway	○	○
Check for breathing (10 seconds)	○	○
Deliver two slow breaths	○	○
Check circulation (carotid pulse 10 seconds)	○	○
CPR initiated until AED is available	○	○
Defibrillation:		
Power is turned on	○	○
Ensure clean/dry skin surface	○	○
Electrodes correctly applied	○	○
Electrode cable plugged in	○	○
Clear victim	○	○
Analyze	○	○
If shock is indicated:		
a. Clear victim	○	○
b. Deliver shock	○	○
c. Analyze	○	○
d. Deliver up to 3 shocks	○	○
e. Pulse check	○	○
f. Perform 1 minute of CPR if no pulse	○	○
g. Analyze	○	○
If shock is indicated repeat steps a–g		
If no shock is indicated:		
Pulse check	○	○
Perform 1 minute of CPR if no pulse	○	○
Analyze	○	○
	Pass	**Fail**